"As a former English teacher, I am keenly aware of the power of words to shape our thoughts and feelings. Meyers offers practical language tweaks for parents and guardians who want to foster a healthy relationship with food and enjoy more peaceful family meals."

—**Oona Hanson, MA, MA**, educator and parent coach, and family mentor at Equip Health

"*End the Mealtime Meltdown* is a unique guide to avoiding food fights with your child. In a calm and reassuring tone, Stephanie Meyers provides tips, tools, and strategies that make eating with kids more peaceful for everyone involved. Meyers's Table Talk Method replaces parental prodding and cajoling with an open communication style that lays the foundation for a child's healthy relationship with food now, and in the future."

—**Elizabeth Ward, MS, RDN**, author of *Expect the Best*

"One of the most important things I've learned from this book is that helping kids have a healthy relationship with food involves encouraging curiosity around new and different types of food. Stephanie shows you how engaging your children with questions around the way ingredients look, taste, or feel can be a gateway to having them accept that food."

—**Leigh Belanger**, author of *My Kitchen Chalkboard*

T0000676

"Where was this thoughtful book twenty years ago when I was raising my kids? This much-needed resource should be on every parent's and grandparent's reading list to prepare for the years of joyful family mealtime gatherings ahead of them. Food should be loved, embraced, and enjoyed, and Meyers nailed it in this soon-to-be classic for raising healthy eaters."

—**Joan Salge Blake, EdD, RDN, FAND**, Boston University
     nutrition professor; author; media personality; and host of
     the nutrition and health podcast, *Spot On!*

"For parents who are committed to raising a generation of healthy eaters, this is an important tool! The book provides creative, stress-free techniques for reducing common but frustrating food struggles at mealtimes. Her practical advice and realistic expectations show parents how to effectively communicate with children to create enjoyable, peaceful mealtimes at last!"

—**Susan Albers, PsyD**, psychologist, and New York Times
     bestselling author of *Eating Mindfully, 50 Ways to Soothe
     Yourself Without Food, Eating Mindfully for Teens*, and
     Hanger Management

"Refreshing and revolutionary! This book is a gift for families as it brings joy, curiosity, and connection back to mealtime. Stephanie Meyers's approach is brilliant—grounded in evidence and practical experience—weaving together her deep knowledge of nutrition counseling, mindfulness, and parenting to break old, unhelpful habits and replace them with new, healthy ways of relating and eating that can last a lifetime."

—**Susan Bauer-Wu, PhD, RN**, president of the
     Mind & Life Institute, and author of *Leaves Falling Gently*

END THE
MEALTIME
MELTDOWN

Using the Table Talk Method to
Free Your Family from Daily Struggles
over Food and Picky Eating

STEPHANIE MEYERS, MS, RDN

New Harbinger Publications, Inc.

Publisher's Note

NEW HARBINGER PUBLICATIONS is a registered trademark of New Harbinger Publications, Inc.

New Harbinger Publications is an employee-owned company.

Distributed in Canada by Raincoast Books

Copyright © 2022 by Stephanie Meyers
New Harbinger Publications, Inc.
5674 Shattuck Avenue
Oakland, CA 94609
www.newharbinger.com

"The Basic Mindful Eating Meditation" is reprinted with permission, from Mindful Eating (2009) by Jan Chozen Bays.

"Ellen Satter's Division of Responsibility in Feeding" is reprinted with permission.

Cover design by Amy Daniel; Acquired by Jess O'Brien; Edited by Brady Kahn

All Rights Reserved

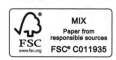

Library of Congress Cataloging-in-Publication Data

Names: Meyers, Stephanie, author.
Title: End the mealtime meltdown : using the table talk methoutrd to free your family from daily struggles over food and picky eating / Stephanie Meyers, MS, RDN.
Description: Oakland : New Harbinger Publications, 2022. | Includes bibliographical references.
Identifiers: LCCN 2021057648 | ISBN 9781684039463 (trade paperback)
Subjects: LCSH: Children--Nutrition. | Children--Nutrition--Psychological aspects.
Classification: LCC RJ206 .M684 2022 | DDC 613.2083--dc23/eng/20211221
LC record available at https://lccn.loc.gov/2021057648

Printed in the United States of America

24   23   22

10   9   8   7   6   5   4   3   2   1   First Printing

To Michael, Hava, and Solin.
Being at the table with you feeds my soul.

Contents

Foreword

I once got into a power struggle with my daughter over a bite of quinoa. I don't mean a spoonful of quinoa. I mean an individual grain. If you have never looked at a single grain of quinoa, it's miniscule—far too small for my daughter to actually taste but apparently not too small for me to overlook in my ongoing quest to get my toddlers to try new foods. Needless to say, it wasn't one of my finer parenting moments.

Thankfully, our food-related power struggles have decreased significantly over the past decade. But I still find myself nagging, bribing, bargaining, and counting bites with my tween-age daughters more often than I'd like to admit. I know these strategies are ineffective, but when my brain starts worrying about the girls' health and eating habits, I don't know what else to do.

At least, I didn't until I heard about Stephanie Meyers' brilliant concept of table talk. This book is unlike any other one I've read on the topic of feeding children—and I've read a lot of them! Meyers doesn't offer advice on how to craft the perfect meal or sneak vegetables into meatloaf. She doesn't scare readers with statistics about childhood obesity and the risk of eating disorders. And thankfully, Meyers doesn't shame or blame parents who are struggling to raise healthy children in a culture that demands perfection while inundating us with contradictory messages about what and how to feed kids.

Rather, Meyers draws on her vast professional and personal experience as a nutritionist and mother to provide readers a simple, straightforward plan that will dramatically change the dynamic at your family table—for the better. Amazingly enough, it doesn't involve a single recommendation as to what we should feed our kids. Rather, Meyers focuses on how we interact with our children. By changing the way we talk to them about what they're eating, while they're eating, we can transform their relationship with food and end the painful power struggles.

Rather than harassing our kids about their food, readers are encouraged to engage their children with questions and prompts such as "What do you notice?" and "Tell me about…" Each time we make space for growing eaters to get curious about their food and connect with their experience of it, we're disabling their defensiveness and supporting their budding gastronomic intelligence—their inner wisdom and awareness of eating. Fortunately for those of us who get stressed, confused, or overwhelmed by the mere mention of gastronomic intelligence, Meyers provides us with a clear plan for precisely how to proceed.

After reading about the Table Talk Method, I found myself moving from a place of reactive, anxiety-fueled comments and suggestions to a calmer, more curious way of speaking to my kids about the food on their plates. By exploring my daughters' eating experience with them, I'm supporting them in trying new foods and finding foods they enjoy, as Meyers notes, "to break up frenetic energy and nip meltdowns in the bud." Each time I'm tempted to remind my girls that they didn't even try their salmon and they might actually like it this time—a tactic which has never once worked in the history of my parenting experience—I can ask them what they're noticing, what's not working for them, and what might help. Instead of nagging my girls to try just one more bite of chicken or rice, I can ask them what their plan is for the food left on their plate, which unused food we should keep, and how we might use it later. Instead of triggering a tense negotiation over every bite, I'm learning to empower my daughters to make intentional choices rather than reactive decisions. And I'm learning to do the same for myself along the way.

If you're looking for wise, evidence-based practices for how to ease food conflict in your family, you've come to the right place. No matter how old your children are, the Table Talk Method will help you move past whatever mealtime dynamic you're stuck in. It will give you the insight and strategies you need to create a culture of curiosity and connection each time you gather around the table, and it will give your children the skills they need for a lifetime of healthy eating.

—Carla Naumburg, PhD, LICSW
Author of *How to Stop Losing Your Sh*t with Your Kids*

CHAPTER 1

Feeling "Down in the Mouth" at Dinner?

The vegetables are sizzling, the rice is steaming, and your family is seated at the table. You've worked all day, driven carpool, and produced a home-cooked meal. No wonder you're triggered when the first thing muttered is "YUCK! We're having stir-fry for dinner?"

Despite feeling irked, you stay calm and say, "Why don't you give it a try? You might like it this time." This yields silent stares. Sighing, you load your own fork and think, *If they're hungry enough, they'll eat it.* Minutes later the rice is gone, but everything else on your child's plate remains untouched. You know the lines by heart.

Parent: Try a little stir-fry. It's delicious! It tastes just like the one you like from *Bamboo.*

Child: I don't want stir-fry. What else can I have?

Parent: This is dinner. Please eat now, because there's not going to be a snack later.

Child: What?! All I get is *rice?*

Parent: And stir-fry.

Child: But I hate stir-fry.

Parent: You didn't even touch it. Just take a bite of chicken *or* vegetables, please.

Child: (*Moaning.*) I don't liiike stir-fry.

Parent: You don't need to like it. I just wish you'd try. You haven't eaten any vegetables all day.

Dinner ends on a sour note, and you brace for what's coming later. Your final plea as your child stomps away: "Did you eat enough?" *No response.* "Remember I said no snack later."

And so it goes, night after night. A helpless and disempowered feeling during meals, for both you and your child. Food and feelings are deeply intertwined, but parenthood takes that to another level. When kids don't eat well, parents feel bad. Not just a little bad. An injurious sense-of-responsibility-and-failure kind of bad. If this is happening to you, you're not alone. A 2016 survey conducted by C.S. Mott Children's Hospital in Michigan found 97 percent of parents believe healthy eating during childhood has a lifelong impact, yet only one in six rate their child's diet as "very healthy" (C. S. Mott Children's Hospital 2017).

Parents are frustrated by what their kids eat and don't eat. They're worried their child will never branch out and try new foods. They're discouraged because the try-new-foods tactics they relied on quit working when their kids hit grade school. They're concerned that their kids "terrible diet" could negatively affect health, growth, and body image or self-esteem. And scrolling social media slaps on more pressure, showcasing kid meals made by food stylists.

Pressure and stress about how kids eat is a problem parents aren't sure how to solve. Only 34 percent of parents feel confident that they're doing a good job of shaping their child's eating habits (C. S. Mott Children's Hospital 2017). Prioritizing and juggling healthy eating is challenging, and crummy feelings about how kids eat can pile up over months and years. One mom described her nine-year grind to improve how her kids eat as "So lousy and confusing, I don't know who's having the bigger meltdown, me or my kids?!"

The ideas in this book are meant to help with the widespread eating challenges parents face, like kids whining about what's for dinner, rejecting vegetables repeatedly, and begging for sweets nonstop. Instead of more mind-numbing advice to "include your child in food shopping," "avoid pressure," and "make mealtime a positive experience," I'll teach you what to say so you're not caught in food negotiations with your kids, whether they are three years old and melting down over food or preteens just buying what they want to eat anyway.

Bad feelings about how your kid eats are common, but here's the rub: something you're doing is working against you. And it's right on the tip of your tongue. I refer to this as *table talk*.

What Is Table Talk?

What I call *table talk* is what you say to your child *about* their eating *while* they're eating. Phrases like "You already had two muffins today," "Stop using your hands!" or "One more bite, then you can be done." For now, think of table talk in two flavors: helpful and unhelpful (we'll get to the specifics later). The Table Talk Method in this book teaches you how to move from ineffective (*old table talk*) to more effective (*new table talk*), because old table talk is the untapped, unexamined root of where things go wrong with feeding kids. It's language we use repeatedly without realizing what those words do.

Table talk happens during meals and snacks, although it's not only confined to those times. It also creeps up just before and after meals in the form of food negotiations. Things like who-wants-this-versus-that, how-much, and "Are you even eating it?" interactions at meals. And don't forget before-bedtime snacks! Table talk looms large in the evening hours.

Table talk includes comments about food and your child's eating behaviors, but it's not only words that wrangle or redirect. It also includes utterances of appreciation and praise like "Thank you for trying this" and "What a good eater!" Table talk is a whole style of language parents and caregivers use with kids around eating that feeds into the unpleasant feelings you face when feeding kids.

Here are some examples of common table talk:

"Take two more bites if you want dessert."

"Good job eating all your broccoli!"

"You liked lasagna last week!"

"But you didn't even *try* it! Please, just take one bite."

"You can't say you don't like it until you try it."

"Don't use your fingers—I gave you a fork."

"That's enough pasta. You need to eat some vegetables too."

"If you eat good food, you'll be strong."

"I'm so proud of you for trying new foods!"

Table talk is the nuts and bolts of our eating interactions with kids. These phrases, sprinkled throughout mealtime, contribute to your child's relationship with food. Even if your child shuns vegetables or eats sloppily today, you have the power with what you say to help change that. How you coach your child's process of eating is the key to less conflict around food. As parents, we shoulder a significant responsibility in the pursuit of raising healthy, happy eaters. Teaching kids how and what to eat is only one piece of the puzzle. Helping them know and trust themselves as eaters is a much bigger deal. Showing them how to relate to food and their body in healthy ways is one of the most important life skills we can impart as parents. But what's a reliable recipe for coaching how kids eat? And what can you do when things aren't going well?

My ideas on how to handle these things evolved from the nexus of four things: my jobs as a mom, a dietitian, and a professor, and my daily meditation practice. At Boston University, I teach graduate students nutrition-counseling skills, things like conscious communication, non-judgment, and active listening, so they learn to cocreate lasting behavior change with clients. Outside the classroom, I see people in my private practice, and I direct nutrition at Dana-Farber Cancer Institute's Integrative Therapies and Healthy Living Center. Conversations with tens of thousands of clients deeply informed my approach, but nothing compelled me on this topic more than becoming a parent myself.

When my oldest daughter was two years old, I had a revelation. Many things I tell students never to say to clients are the very phrases that parents dish out to kids while they eat. I began exploring what I labeled *table talk* through the lens of my own parenting (gulp), my mindfulness practice, and my experience as a nutritionist. I surveyed parents nationwide, gathering anonymous submissions of table talk, and led focus groups about the challenges parents face feeding their kids. I listened carefully to parent-child interactions around food and considered my clients' narratives from an entirely new perspective. I took a long, hard look at moments I was goading my own kids with food. My observations led to new ways of parenting the process of kids eating well, which I call the Table Talk Method. I'm excited to teach it to you, because it brings more peace and joy to family moments around food.

The scientific underpinnings of my work include research on mindful eating, relational communications, and childhood development around food. My ideas are based on evidence about how kids make food choices, how parents prompt kids to eat, and how behavior change happens in humans. I won't go in-depth on the literature here, but it's worth noting that many parental feeding practices lead to lower vegetable intake and pickier eating (Jordan et al. 2020; Jansen et al. 2017). We also know kids grow up internalizing messages from others around eating (Ogden and Roy-Stanley 2020), and experiences of childhood feeding (as studied in mother-daughter dyads) have a lasting impact on how kids eat as adults (Roberts et al. 2020).

If that's too much to absorb, never mind what the research says. I want to focus on training you with new skills that bring about better eating outcomes for your kid. By learning new skills (like open-ended questions), you will help your child gain new skills (like exploring new foods without pressure). Food and eating are complex behaviors, but the resources you need to make things better are something you have within.

How to Use This Book

The Table Talk Method works best for parents of kids ages two to twelve, and while it's nice to start early, your child's age is not a limiting factor. Sometimes parents of older kids worry that entrenched ways of eating over years means they won't benefit from changing how they talk with their kids. In my experience, it's the opposite. Parents who use this new approach with kids age eight and up find their kids have the vocabulary and verbal skills to go deep with new table talk. Besides, the older your child gets, the more sophisticated they become at taking issue with what you think and say about their eating. This means anytime is a great time to start revamping how you talk with your child about their eating. It's a doorway to improving the quality of how and what they eat and their long-term relationship with food.

Before we go further, eating issues—even in kids—come in different varieties and extremes. This book does not address or serve as a replacement for professional medical advice on sensory-related eating problems or extreme picky eating. A pediatrician, board-certified speech-language pathologist, and registered dietitian specializing in eating or feeding therapy are the best resources for guidance on these problems. The scope of this book does not include treating kids or families with eating disorders such as anorexia nervosa, bulimia nervosa, and avoidant restrictive food intake disorder (ARFID). For help with these issues, please contact a qualified medical professional.

This book is about self-discovery. It is not about memorizing lines but about reimagining how you relate to your child over food. You'll personalize what you learn through writing exercises, which means you'll need a separate notebook or journal. Nothing fancy, just a consistent place to write things down and refer to over time. There are also some materials available for download at the website for this book: http://www. newharbinger.com/49463. (See the very back of this book for more details.)

The eating challenges you face today are top priority here, so the exercises and journal entries are important to do. They help you customize things to suit your needs. We'll work together with pen, paper, and your voice to improve eating in your family and to release you from the stress and guilt that can come with feeding kids. The ideas I share are not just things I teach but values I live and practice every day. If you think things will never change with how your child eats, I understand. Together, we'll create a whole new menu of effective things to say.

Check In with Yourself

How often do you say the same thing over and over with no measurable improvement in your child's eating behaviors or food acceptance patterns? Typical table talk doesn't lead to the results we hope for as parents. And even when it does (when your kid eats what you ask them to eat), how you got there might not be something you want to repeat. For example, "Some kids don't have enough food…" is clean-plate club propaganda that you might've sworn off. But in a desperate moment when your kid just won't eat, it slips your lips and you get a rush of guilt at the table.

Typical table talk is familiar and disquieting, featuring repetitive instructions and unsavory demands like begging, bribing, and pleading. Most of that language is a means to an end. But what is that end? Often it's a bad feeling for both parents and kids. Unexamined table talk adds tension to family meals. It raises the risk that rotten feelings will come up, and it brings on food-centered meltdowns. And typical table talk not only affects how kids eat but also exacerbates your stress level as a parent.

But don't take it from me that your table talk is making you feel lousy. The point of doing the work in this book is to test it out in your own life! Practice using the new words you learn, even if they sound weird at first. Approaching these ideas with an open mind gives you the most mileage toward improving family dynamics around food. Some things will stick more than others. Take what helps and leave the rest. The Table Talk Method adapts with your family over time, so even if something doesn't click right away, you can try it again later. The goal is to learn how to coach your child's eating in new and intentional ways that feel and work better for both you and them. I don't believe there's only one right way to do this, and so I encourage you to try these ideas in situations where you feel caught up or stuck in parenting around food.

When you think about how table talk shows up in your daily life, you might feel like you need it, like it's an essential part of how you stay "in charge" or manage things during meals. Kids can be erratic with food, and what you say is something you honestly hope will help them get along better with eating. Typical table talk is meant to be effective, but it routinely fails, because qualities like self-trust and ownership around eating are things kids must develop for themselves. Add to that a sense of satisfaction, worthiness, and self-compassion around food, and you've got a list of important things you might desire yourself, not to mention hope to teach your kids, about eating. Typical table talk impedes that process. Understanding and upgrading what you say to your child as they eat teaches them vital skills around food while it simultaneously opens new doors for true cooperation at your family table.

What is cooperation over food? Cooperation is working together to get something done, and when that something is eating well—or even eating at all—it takes parents and kids banding together. Ending conflict at mealtime isn't about getting your kid straightened out with food. It's not "overcoming pickiness" or expecting compliance with eating. It's working in collaboration with your child to create new possibilities at the table—the very possibilities we usually pass over due to what we say during meals.

Consider Your Kid's Experience

Most young kids don't buy their own food. They don't plan or cook their meals, at least not by themselves. They eat or refuse whatever comes to the table—at school, at home, or on the sidelines. Sounds simple, right? But it's not. Kids have desires, delights, and disgusts when it comes to food. They have sight, smell, texture, temperature, and flavor preferences and aversions. What they lack is sovereignty in eating situations.

They probably didn't purchase, choose, or prepare what's on their plate, yet they're awash in sensations, thoughts, and feelings about that food, whether they eat it or not. A symphony of experiences unfolds in each kid's mind and body as they eat. And as parents, we're talking— table talking—when what's really called for is listening. The problem with usual table talk is that it doesn't activate what kids really need as eaters: cues and the chance to explore, observe, process, and honor what's happening with food and eating in the moment.

Most of the language we use when coaching kids to eat is instructive rather than inquisitive. Typical table talk is full of directions about what we want kids to do. *Eat more, slow down, take smaller bites,* and *focus on eating.* But children need less admonishment and more exploration while eating, along with the acknowledgment that what they notice about food is valuable information.

Eating Well Is a Learned Skill

It makes sense to repeat detailed instructions when teaching kids certain skills like tying shoes or brushing teeth. For these tasks, routine guidance trains kids to get the job done. Persistent verbal cues help kids tweak technique and master these skills, eventually enabling a kind of automation in their life. For other skills, however, directive language isn't the best fit. It doesn't help kids develop autonomy and self-reliance. Eating is this second type of skill.

As a toddler, my daughter was obsessed with Os—not the breakfast cereal but the letter. Stiffening excitedly, she'd point and holler, "O!" at STOP signs and at oatmeal containers. But the thrill of spotting Os was a recognition beyond the letter. Those "Look mom!" moments fed her tender sense of belonging. No mind to the twenty-five other letters she had yet to discover—she was worthy and connected, partaking in the great big world around her.

Kids acquire life skills from this wide-eyed place of wonder, and we nurture that development by capitalizing on their curiosity. This unfolds naturally when teaching kids to read. There's a bouncy tune for the alphabet and lilting chants ("C, cat, ck,"), to teach sounds. Parents and teachers use specific practices to help kids advance from simple syllables to sophisticated stories. It's a gradual process where adults use basic tools with consistent goodwill. All of this has crossover potential for how we coach kids to eat.

Coaching kids to eat well is like helping them learn to read, except we rarely approach it that way. Reading we view as a process, expecting imperfections along the way. We believe it takes years to become proficient, and we strive to keep advancing over a lifetime. We accept that learning to read involves many steps and struggles, and we face those situations with a certain savoir faire. Teaching literary skills to kids is effortful and exacting, yet somehow the day-to-day operations come off very differently from teaching kids to eat well.

Consider when kids write their Ss backwards. At first, it's kind of cute, but we know (and trust) at some point they'll turn things around. We don't expect conformity or criticize their tongue-jutting efforts to get it straight. And when kids mostly master Ss, we practice patience for the Js. Drilling kids to squiggle "S" correctly takes a backseat to maintaining their interest and enthusiasm for the process. Imagine employing these attitudes when coaching kids to eat!

Appreciating new flavors and foods takes time and practice much like learning the shapes and sounds of letters. But we seldom approach it that way. Take a kid who hates broccoli, for example. What if a child's resistance to broccoli was dealt with like a backwards S? How can we rethink broccoli fiascos to account for effort? Maybe kids need new ways of acquainting with broccoli? Sometimes they make a good effort. How do we acknowledge that?

When a child writes the letter S backwards, we don't say, "You need to at least try the Ss. You can't leave the table until you try three more." Substitute "broccoli" for "Ss" in that statement, however, and it's a painfully precise snippet of what we say to kids about eating. How we interact with kids around food is profoundly different from how we teach other life skills. Once you recognize this, you can change it for good. You've got more on the shelf right now than you realize to help your child eat well. I'll give you lots of new skills and help you reinvigorate some old skills that might be lying dormant.

If You're Feeling Wary

I also want to be clear that focusing on table talk isn't meant to make you feel bad about yourself or what you've said to your kids during meals. In fact, this process involves learning to consciously let those feelings be, so you can break the cycle and adopt new skills that infuse curiosity and autonomy at the table. The Table Talk Method is not about identifying shortcomings in your parenting around food but about tapping into the unrecognized wellspring of capacity that you already possess. It's not choking back your words for fear of saying something wrong, and it's not ignoring certain behaviors you can't stand at the table.

When kids forgo their napkin, for example, smearing food or grease on their pants, you can address that behavior with clarity of message and intent. But instead of scolding them for the umpteenth time, you'll learn to say only one word—an ING-verb—paired with a demonstration of the action you want your child to take. So "Stop wiping your hands on your pants!" gets transformed to one simple word: "Wiping." You say this word kindly while simultaneously using your napkin to demonstrate the cleaning of hands. Then you move on. The whole thing takes three seconds. And two minutes later, when your child wipes their mouth on their sleeve, you simply repeat the process. Say one ING-verb, "Wiping," as you demonstrate using your napkin to wipe your mouth.

Simple tools like using ING-verbs, taught in the Table Talk Method, cause new things to happen. Your kid—yes, even the grade schooler— might start to follow your lead, even if it's just because they're totally perplexed. Omitting your habitual reaction and associated table talk is sometimes enough to capture your kid's attention and prompt a sought-after change. One ING-verb is a gentle word of redirection that replaces all the drama, so no one loses it over the napkin. The other thing that happens with new table talk is you avoid shaming language. You'll hear more about this as we go along, but, in a nutshell, self-compassion brings better results than shame.

If you're thinking *This won't work with my kid,* your skepticism is welcome here. In the Table Talk Method, your doubt is an asset. You can think that this whole concept is absurd and still reap the benefits, because welcoming uncertainty is the name of the game when it comes to feeding kids. I'll show you how to channel your wariness into productive curiosity, but it requires you give things an honest try, not just write them off.

Multiple Benefits Await You

The Table Talk Method not only teaches you what to say when you're provoked by your kids' eating behavior but also works when kids are eating with relative ease. You'll learn effective language to address all kinds of things like manners, food rejection, and concerns about over- or undereating. Above all, you'll learn to nurture the most important things, pleasure, joy, and contentedness around food, without feelings of shame. Transforming your table talk does great things for kids—how they eat and who they are as eaters—while it also relieves some of the angst you might be feeling during meals. To name a few more benefits for kids, implementing new table talk:

- Improves eating habits in the short and long term

- Encourages greater variety and expansion of kids' palettes

- Sparks an interest in trying new foods without feeling pressured

- Fosters a healthy relationship with food and nurtures body confidence

- Strengthens relational bonds between caregivers and kids

- Supports your child's belief in their own abilities around food

- Builds awareness of self-satisfaction, self-trust, and self-compassion around eating

- Eases tension around food resistance and rejection

- Avoids pitfalls of food- and eating-related shame

- Facilitates kids' development as eaters with clear purpose and intent

Changing your table talk works by lifting you out of the struggle. One or two new phrases can change the tune and direction of an entire meal. When table talk invites kids inside their own experience of eating, they don't feel the need to push back. And you're not stuck in fruitless negotiations that leave you feeling bad.

With new words you show your child that there is value in their awareness and insights about eating—that you care about it. This liberates both of you in important ways. For my client Claire, mom of three, it meant, "breaking free from appraising and comparing how my kids eat— out loud in front of everyone." Claire's work on table talk helped her undo entrenched patterns and use better words with her seven-year-old who "doesn't eat enough" and her nine-year-old and thirteen-year-old who "load up on carbs." The Table Talk Method works kid by kid across a wide range of situations, giving you more resilience for the ups and downs of mealtime.

How Table Talk Impacts Your Child

How you interact with your child over food impacts their development as an eater. Table talk is the raw material of how that collaboration unfolds. Words spoken about food and eating become a soundtrack for the inner dialogue kids record as eaters. Table talk phrases can provoke or propel. They can promote or prohibit. And while they're largely unexamined, you have the ability to change them.

What you say to your kid about food and behavior while they eat is important because it's the gateway to engaging their internal cues and awareness of eating. Table talk is how you connect with your kid around food. Your words literally guide your child's self-discovery as an eater, which is why learning to change table talk, where needed, can yield seismic shifts at mealtime.

Why focus on words? Parents who've never heard of table talk still use it every day, if not at every meal. This isn't meant to make you feel guilty; it simply points to the fact that we have lots and lots of opportunities to awaken if we choose. I've never found a guidebook devoted to how we talk with kids about their eating, and I'd never claim to understand all the conditioned and nuanced ways table talk evolves. What I do know is that table talk is deeply habituated and counterintuitive. Rote reminders like "Focus on eating. Your food is getting cold" lead to beseeching, "Can you *please* just take a few bites? You hardly touched your plate."

Despite our best intentions to help kids eat well, much of what we say to them during meals inadvertently botches the job. Table talk is one variable amidst the vagaries of feeding kids that you as a parent have the capacity to control. Learning about table talk and how to change it unlocks paradigm shifts, so you and your child will be happier (and healthier) at the table.

You're Not Doing It All Wrong

There's nothing more offensive than someone implying that your parenting is off track, and that is never my intention. If the table talk examples you find on these pages feel unnervingly familiar, I understand. They do for me too. Every example of table talk I share— especially the cringeworthy ones—are things I've said to my own kids at one time or another. My intent is to support, not criticize, you or your parenting. As a mom myself, I'm intimately familiar with the humbling and, at times, demoralizing process of trying my best, yet falling short on a regular basis. When I critique table talk like "Take two more bites," or "Just try it please," I don't do so through a lens of judgment and superiority. I'm not a parenting expert (is that even a thing?) and I'm not here to finger-wag. I'm parenting right alongside you, in all the rigmarole of feeding a family.

I can't emphasize enough the value of an ongoing personal practice with table talk. This is not a finish line you cross by scripting all the right words but a continuous awakening that happens meal by meal. I developed this method, and I still learn new things every day! I'm a participating parent with a viewpoint and language that I hope feels useful for you. My aim is to help you feel well versed and confident in creating the kind of relationship you seek with your kid around food.

How This Method Differs from Others You've Tried

Parents today are rather sophisticated when it comes to feeding kids. Many utilize Ellyn Satter's approach known as Satter's Division of Responsibility in Feeding (sDOR) (Satter 1986). Satter's delineation of roles for both parents and kids establishes who's in charge of different parts of eating. Parents decide the what, when, and where of food while kids oversee if and how much they eat from what is served. This framework is revolutionary because it confers trust in kids and gives both parents and children clear jobs when it comes to eating.

The sDOR is a model that I urge parents to embrace. If you're new to sDOR, read *Child of Mine* (Satter 2000) for examples of how to apply it in feeding your infant, toddler, and preschooler. You can also refresh your understanding of sDOR by reading the brief overview in the appendix of this book.

The Table Talk Method adds on to the infrastructure Ellyn Satter lays out in sDOR. If you already use sDOR, you can think of the Table Talk Method as a warning system of sorts. It audibly alerts you when you've crossed a division of responsibility line. Parents getting in the wrong DOR lane often happens verbally (vis-a-vis table talk).

Other techniques parents use to help kids eat more or better include "veggie exposure," "food chaining," "tasting plates," and "no-thank-you bowls." Many parents find these strategies helpful to address picky eating behaviors, and they don't need to be abandoned to use the Table Talk Method. In fact, these ideas often work better when parents add new language to the mix, such as wondering, open-ended questions and reflective statements, which you'll learn about in chapter 6.

Parents aren't novices at trying to get kids to eat better. We cut food into cute shapes, strategically placing new foods alongside safe ones. We space foods apart that *absolutely can't touch* and serve vegetables over and over again. We already say, "You don't have to eat it," despite our reticent qualms. *But do they? Shouldn't they? Can we really let them keep skipping whole groups of food they probably need?* This is another place you might feel stuck, not knowing what to do or say after you've already said, "You don't have to eat it," for the hundredth time. Because, the truth is, it doesn't really feel that way sometimes. If you're like most parents, you've tried many things meant to help your kids eat better, but you're still waiting for something to click and wondering what to say in the meantime.

No matter what you've tried to help your kid eat better, it can all fall apart simply with what you say. Take Ben, for example, dad of eight-year-old twins whom he kept patiently serving carrots. He prepared carrots dozens of times in different ways: raw, cooked, even spiralized into noodles, but every attempt was a bust. Then Ben heard about table talk and dug a bit deeper. He found what he was saying was unwittingly thwarting his efforts: questions like "Can you try the star-shaped carrot?" or "Do you want the yummy carrot sauce on top?" These are closed-ended questions, and they're one of eight types of table talk that undermine even the most creative veggie-exposure plans. In chapter 3, we'll break this down, so you understand what old table talk is made of and why it's counterproductive at mealtime.

Despite our advancing knowledge and creativity at the family table, one thing we still haven't effectively addressed is what we say to kids while they eat. It can be hard to hear, but as parents and caregivers, we routinely serve the most wholesome foods with the least helpful phrases. And while changing your table talk isn't the only way to improve your family's food dynamics, it might be the only thing you haven't tried.

A Plan for Change

This book guides you through the process of becoming aware of and transforming your table talk. It helps you identify patterns and unlock new skills to leverage change at your family table. It gives you specific tools to cultivate curiosity, mindful eating, and conscious communication and teaches you how to remodel your words to get unstuck in the process of feeding your family.

Becoming aware of your table talk affords you hidden leeway. That's because you compose and control it, unlike many other parts of eating with kids. In the daily struggle of feeding kids, you might not realize you're up against a wall—a wall that you alone can take down. When you recognize and replace the unintended messages typical table talk conveys, you regain precious bandwidth and have an easier time navigating tough moments with your kids over food.

When parents and caregivers first learn about table talk, they say similar things:

- "I didn't realize what I say to my kids while they eat could make a difference!"

- "I'm embarrassed about what I say (now that I'm listening to my words)."

- "I've had it with all the fussing and whining about food."

- "I say things about eating I'm not proud of, but I'm not sure what else to do."

- "Feeding my kids is so stressful."

- "I don't know what to say to my child to build positive connections with food."

When kids won't eat vegetables today—or this year!—the question isn't how you can make them. It's how you can parent in a more productive way to help them engage with new foods of their own accord. The Table Talk Method is about uncovering a habituated lexicon, examining your table talk, and learning how to change it for the better.

To do this, you'll identify your own table talk, learning to relate to it without judgment. Then you'll work to understand its impact on both you and your child. Next, you'll practice ways of engaging your child with food that *parent their eating process* instead of what's on their plate. Finally, you'll replace old table talk phrases with optimal new table talk, gaining specific language to guide your child's evolution as an eater. The result is more workability for you and your kid, so it's easier to hang in there when there's trouble with food.

The Table Talk Method rests on your willingness to experiment with the hidden power of language and how you relate to your kids while they eat. This approach is accessible to anyone eating with kids, regardless of time or place. Best of all, the new skills you'll learn work long term, so the stuff that's been dragging you down during meals becomes your new way forward.

Mindfully Making New Patterns

The Table Talk Method is a set of practical skills parents use to decrease stress and frustration for everyone in their family. It's swapping out old patterns and phrases in favor of new table talk rooted in mindful eating and conscious communication. The first part of table talk training therefore involves uncovering behaviors and language you may not even realize you use. Cultivating awareness of these things will offer insight into how they impact your child's eating and your stress level as a parent. With a better understanding of your usual table talk and its effects, you can figure out what to say instead.

One thing that's critically important to remember as you do this work is that self-judgment siphons energy you need to reach your goals. And feeling bad about your table talk *does not* deliver a better outcome. So let's focus instead on the takeaways you can expect from cutting old words loose. Parents who use the table talk method gain:

- A mindful eating and communication pathway to engage children in building healthy eating habits for a lifetime

- Specific language prompts that spark kids' willingness to engage with food

- A simple but effective way to manage resistance around food and eating

- A fresh approach and understanding of how to undo old patterns and customize new table talk, so your message aligns with your parenting values around food

- A method that continues to work over the years as kids grow up

This book takes a different tack from other things you might have tried. It's not based on food and nutrition tips. It teaches you how to talk to kids about their eating, so meals are more enjoyable, and they learn to connect with and trust their inner compass around food. Food fiascos end when you move in a new direction, tapping into something I call *gastronomic intelligence* (GI). No worries if that sounds esoteric—I'll teach you all about it in chapter 5. Besides, gastronomic intelligence is something you already have (all humans do!) I'll show you how to access and work with it in a straightforward way. But let's start at the beginning and work our way through.

Your job is to stay honest, come as you are, and do the work from your own experience. You're the expert in what it's like to eat with your kid, so let's get the lowdown on that. This first exercise captures how things are going with feeding your child today and your impressions of healthy eating.

EXERCISE: Defining Healthy Eating

Answer the following questions in your journal. Be as specific as you can.

1. What constitutes "healthy eating" from your perspective? What behaviors define healthy eating in kids? A willingness to try new foods? Expanding the variety or amount of foods eaten? Respectful manners, enjoying food fully, feeling

gratitude? Eating sufficient veggies or avoiding "too much junk?" What else?

2. Circle the things on this list that feel most important to you.

3. If these qualities were thriving in your home, what would that look like? What would be an indication your child was "eating well?"

4. What's your child doing during meals that you hope will change? What are they not doing that you hope improves?

5. What stresses you out the most about feeding your kid(s) these days?

With this information in hand, it's time to take a closer look at your table talk.

Feeding kids can feel like a low point in parenting, but you're on the brink of a new discovery: what you say to your child over food is a powerful change maker. Adopting new language helps your child eat better while lowering your stress level during meals. The first step is taking inventory of your current table talk and exploring it.

CHAPTER 2

Take Inventory of Your Table Talk

Ten-year-old Tina played piano with a paper cup of green beans at her side. She failed to finish her veggies at dinner, so her mom scraped them up and handed them over with a polite request, "Please finish these while you practice."

Tina is an adult now, but she still feels a twinge of dread around green beans and certain sonatas. She sympathizes, however, with her mom's intentions now that she's a parent herself. Tina doesn't use Dixie cups or force food to be finished, but she struggles getting her three kids (ages twelve, seven, and five) to eat vegetables. Every day, Tina uses kind and demure table talk like "Your taste buds are always changing. Maybe you'll like green beans next time you try?" But she's frustrated because her efforts to serve healthy food and choose her words carefully aren't helping anyone in her family face the beans.

Tina started exploring table talk because she wanted a different way of relating to her kids around food. Her childhood memories about eating fed lifelong feelings that compel her to parent with intention during meals. Tina is like many parents I work with. She knows a lot about food. She's a member of online groups sharing recipes and strategies to get kids to try more or new foods, but she describes "hitting a wall" with these ideas once her kids reached a certain age.

Tina's breakthrough happened as she was collecting her own table talk. She found a new entry point for connecting with her kids over food. She recalls, "I was swimming in unhelpful table talk, not realizing what it was doing to us at meals! Changing what I say has given me better options when my kids go to pieces at dinner."

In this chapter, I'll lead you through a gentle investigation of what you say to your own kid about their food and eating behaviors, as you take inventory of your table talk. By way of reminder, table talk can happen before, during, or after meals or snacks and at other times too. Table talk is a universal part of parenting. Everyone uses it, and your goal is not to get rid of it but to learn a more helpful version. Table talk around food tends to be knee-jerk and reflexive. This means when you listen for it on purpose, what you say might try to morph. You'll know this is happening when you start fumbling for words midsentence while talking to your child about their food or eating. They'll get up to their usual antics, and suddenly you're tripping on words looking for something "better" to say. Don't try to autocorrect your table talk or avoid saying something you think might be wrong. Right now, your task is just noticing, not changing or judging your words.

Again, your table talk doesn't make you a bad parent. Shining a light on these words, especially in the beginning, can dredge up feelings of parental inadequacy, but if this happens to you, you're not alone, and you're not doing anything wrong. Table talk is ubiquitous in parenting, and looking at it can make you feel self-conscious and exposed. It's worth it, though, because transforming your table talk empowers you to help your kids with food in a way that honors their development as eaters.

If you didn't know table talk existed until twenty pages ago, or you're suddenly swimming in a sea of regret, go easy on yourself. Set bad feelings aside, so you can gain the leverage you need to make food struggles less prominent in your life. The relief you seek is within reach for both you and your kids.

Your Personal Table Talk Inventory

It's time to take inventory of your current table talk. This is your first step toward resolving food conflict. As you gather phrases, be gracious toward yourself. There will be days, meals, snacks, or bedtimes when you'd rather not write down what you say. Don't edit or omit the tough stuff, however, because this approach includes help with nonjudgment. If you're feeling guilty right now, don't close the book. Hang with me through this chapter, and rest assured, we'll discuss coping with self-blame about table talk throughout the book. Your goal is to unearth, not attack, your words.

The purpose of this table talk inventory is to become aware of your current language, not to scrutinize yourself or a partner in the process. Table talk is conditioned and mechanical, so plucking it from thin air and putting it on paper helps you see it more clearly. Table talk phrases in print also help you identify themes and get a general sense if what you're saying matches your intentions around food.

Working Alone or with a Partner

You can do this exercise alone or with a partner if you choose. It doesn't have to be a spouse or coparent. A trusted friend, family member, or any adult who eats with you and your child will be suitable. If you do this exercise with a partner, I recommend you both agree to these rules of engagement in advance:

1. Write table talk down just as it's spoken. Don't add commentary about what was said.

2. No keeping score, or trying to decide who's the bigger table talk offender.

3. Refrain from offering constructive feedback or suggestions of any kind. Don't try to "fix" what your partner says.

The purpose of this exercise is gathering your table talk without adding layers of judgment.

EXERCISE: Your Current Table Talk

This exercise is in two parts. You'll need your journal and a pen for both parts.

Part 1

This part of the exercise takes five minutes. After a brief self-guided visualization, you'll answer six short prompts. When it's time to write, don't change your comments to sound like something you think you should say. Just record precisely what you would say to your child in that moment.

Write "My Current Table Talk" at the top of a blank page in your journal where you'll respond to the prompts. Now think of one food your child doesn't like—something they predictably reject. Keep this food in mind and use it in place of "X" when you do the self-guided visualization and respond to the prompts. For example, if your child doesn't eat asparagus, you would substitute "asparagus" for each X when you write your responses in your journal.

Self-guided visualization: Imagine having dinner with your child. You're sitting at the table with your own plate of food before you. Notice X on your child's plate—it's untouched. Feel your presence beside your child. Take in the sight, smell, and sense of being together.

Imagine your child starts fussing about X. Let the story come alive in your mind. What is your child doing to show resistance to X? Whining? Crying? Using words of disgust? Pushing their plate away? Keep this image of your child rejecting X in your mind.

Now envision your child saying the following things. (If your child is too young to talk, you can pretend for now). Take one phrase at a time, and write down what you would say to your child in response. Don't overthink it. Just answer honestly.

What do you say when your child says this?

1. "I don't like X."

2. "I don't want X."

3. "I *hate* X!"

4. "I don't like X anymore."

5. "Why do we ALWAYS have to eat X?"

6. "But I *did* try X, and I still don't like it!"

Now that you've recorded your perceived table talk, it's time to pay attention to what you actually say.

Part 2

Over the next week, write down your table talk in real time. Keep your journal or some sticky notes handy to jot things down right away. Table talk left undocumented tends to flee the mind fast, so writing it down as soon as you can gets the best results. You'll hear phrases that didn't come up in the visualization. That's good! It means you're capturing a more complete picture of your table talk.

Some parents want to record table talk using their phone. I discourage this for two reasons: it makes kids think you're up to something (they might feel self-conscious or judged), and you need to write your table talk down anyway to do the work ahead. If you record table talk, please do it discreetly and transpose your quotes in your journal as soon as you can. Recording table talk that you never listen to again won't help you make progress. Remember to capture table talk at snacks and unplanned eating intervals in addition to meals. Write down as many phrases as you can in the coming week.

Enlisting a partner while you collect table talk can be advantageous because it's easier to hear another person's table talk than it is to catch your own. You might notice certain table talk that doesn't register for your partner and vice versa, which helps you cast the widest net possible for catching table talk phrases. As you do this exercise, be sure to record your table talk for at least a week, citing as many examples as you can. If you're doing this exercise with partner, add whatever table talk they hear you use to the list you've started in your journal. What you compile will enable you to transform how you talk to your kids during meals.

A friendly reminder to not judge yourself or your words as you complete this process. This isn't about finding fault with the table talk you record. You'll redesign these words soon anyway, so they're basically dust in the wind. For now, just get your table talk down on paper without criticism.

Once you're collecting table talk, you might have some questions about what counts. Let's take a minute to get clear on that, so your inventory is as useful as possible.

What Counts as Table Talk?

Table talk is anything you say to your child about their food and eating habits or behaviors. Table talk is usually spoken to kids while they eat but can also happen in moments just before or after eating. For example, when your child is clamoring for a snack and you say, "Enough pretzels. We're about to have dinner!" that counts as table talk. Snack negotiations between meals or at bedtime are also table talk. When in doubt, write it down. We'll sort through it later.

Here are some examples of a table talk inventory from parents of kids age six and nine.

"This is what's for dinner."

"You've eaten it before and liked it."

"I made it just how you like."

"If you want to be strong and fast…"

"Can you please just try one bite?"

"That's enough chips."

"You didn't even taste it."

"You haven't even touched your plate! Come on…it's time to eat!"

"Take two more bites of this, or you'll have to skip dessert tonight."

"You need to eat at least half of that before you leave the table."

"Thanks for at least giving it a try!"

Note that table talk doesn't always sound incriminating. For example, it may include words of appreciation and praise, such as "Good job eating your broccoli!" or "I'm proud of you for trying that!" Include in your inventory any and all phrases you say, without labeling them good or bad.

Now would be a good time to pause. You may want to bookmark this page as you take time to collect your table talk. It's not mandatory to stop reading here, but don't skip recording phrases, because you're going to need that data later.

If you're opening the book again after a pause to collect table talk, *start here*.

With your table talk phrases in hand, it's time to reflect on what you've gathered. The next exercise will help you get a sense of how table talk is affecting you.

EXERCISE: How Table Talk Makes You Feel

Open your journal to the list of table talk quotes you've gathered so far.

1. Circle the table talk phrases in your journal that you say most often.

2. Underline the table talk phrases that "work" in the sense that your child eats as you say.

3. Put a star next to the phrases that accurately represent your parenting values around food or eating. Star things you hope your child *feels* or *believes* about food and eating.

Looking at your quotes, are the ones you underlined also circled and starred? It's not about how many marks you made but about how you feel about these phrases. On the next page in your journal, respond to these questions:

- Is your table talk all equal, or do some phrases feel more charged?

- What judgments are you making of the situation? About your table talk and yourself?

- Is what you say to your kid while they eat making meals easier?

- Does your table talk smooth out food-related conflict?

- Does what you say give you confidence or set you up to feel bad?

Your answers to these questions pinpoint where you're at now, and they preview where we're headed. You're on track to adopt new language that will help your child eat better, not leave you feeling bad, and capture what you want to teach your child about food and eating.

Seeing your table talk on paper (with or without stars!) can lead to self-critical commentary. When judgments like that come up, view them as clouds passing in the sky. They're not here to stay. Releasing language that's working against you means taking stock of phrases without taking them personally as a parent. No matter what you've been saying, you haven't ruined your chances to help your child eat better. Your willingness to explore how you relate to them while they eat means you're already on a new path—one that I hope will release you from guilt and frustration around food.

A Fresh Start Each Time

Eating always happens in the present. You can *remember* eating, and you can also *imagine* eating, but the grub only really goes down right here in the moment. That means whatever table talk flies out of your mouth, it's over and done. Rehashing old words you wish you hadn't said won't help you move forward, and worrying about future table talk is futile because that moment isn't here yet. The upshot is that any (and every!) moment of eating is your fresh start.

Being free of judgment around table talk involves learning to stay in the moment, because the present moment perpetually gives you the chance to begin again. Nonjudgment also includes forgiving yourself when you say something you regret. In coming chapters you'll learn what to do and say when things go sideways during meals. I'll teach you how to check in and figure out what you meant to convey. Then, in real time, you'll redo your table talk to more accurately capture your feelings and intent. You'll practice this regularly (many times each day), because there's no such thing as perfect table talk. Or perfect parenting.

Many parents report positive side-effects from table talk training. They get more in tune with themselves around food because of what they learn to say to their kids. Part of the Table Talk Method is about deepening these very connections, between you and your child and between your child and their food and lived experiences while eating. It doesn't mean having no problems at the table, but when problems do come up, you won't be left drifting. You'll have new tools, greater flexibility, and a wider range of possible responses.

In the next chapter, we'll dissect typical table talk and compare your words to things commonly said. In preparation for that, pull out your journal once more.

EXERCISE: Explore Nine Principles of the Table Talk Method

As you read each of the following statements, note whether it is *true* or *false* for you. These statements introduce nine cognitive and heart-centered principles of the Table Talk Method.

1. *I am committed to improving how I interact with my child around food.* True or false?

2. *Examining what I say to my kids as they eat, and how it impacts eating behavior, is a new idea for me.* True or false?

3. *Table talk is a universal part of parenting, even if I didn't know about it before.* True or false?

4. *Training on how to talk to my kids about eating isn't something I have received.* True or false?

5. *What I say to my child while they're eating comes from a place of wanting what's best for them even if I have not been taught what to say.* True or false?

6. *Better table talk isn't about perfect phraseology; it's a shift in both mindset and words to engage with my child differently while they eat.* True or false?

7. *When I use table talk that I later regret, I will let go of self-criticism and start anew in the moment.* True or false?

8. *No one meal, snack, treat, or comment represents the totality of my child's eating.* True or false?

9. *When I judge what I say to my kids about eating, I'll remember I'm not doing it all wrong. No parent is doing everything right.* True or false?

There are no right or wrong answers here, but I hope these concepts resonate with you and help you access your inner wisdom and capacity as a parent. From here, you're ready to sort through your table talk.

You have taken inventory of your words and mindset and are about to chart a new course. To do that, I'll give you a tour of common table talk and help you hear how it lands. We'll zoom out from your own words to get a bird's-eye view of typical table talk, which means you can let everything you've done so far just rest for a while. I'll teach you the eight main types of typical table talk and their potential implications. Then you'll consider how that relates to your personal table talk ways.

CHAPTER 3

Typical Table Talk Styles

The table was set, the lasagna and salads served, with three of the four in our family chomping away. But not my five-year-old daughter. Wrinkling her nose in disgust, she twisted and turned with "chair-nastics" activity. That is, she executed gymnastics maneuvers in the confines of a dining room chair. If you're five years old, chair-nastics is a great way to avoid eating salad.

My mood shifted instantaneously, giving way to my unbridled thought reel: *She hasn't eaten a green vegetable in days! What's going on? She usually loves salads! How am I going to get her to eat right now? Ugh! All that junk food from parties this weekend! What's she doing with that leg?!*

Suddenly, I snapped to, remembering my modus operandi is helping parents figure out what to do and say in precisely this type of situation. Table talk phrases blew through my mind. Stuff that never works, but gets repeated anyway, like:

- "Focus on eating. This isn't time for gymnastics."

- "Can you please eat some salad?"

- "Why aren't you eating your salad?"

- "If you don't eat salad, you won't be ready for lasagna."

- "But I made it just how you like—with croutons?!"

Dodging those old standards, I coughed this up instead: "Eat some salad, so you'll be strong for gymnastics."

As soon as I said it, I wanted to eat my words. My intention was good, but my table talk was ineffectual. I told my daughter to eat (now) to cause something desirable to happen (later). This if-then approach to eating, which I call *conditional table talk*, is one of eight types of problematic language I've identified through my work with parents over the years. In this chapter, I'll introduce you to these eight types of typical table talk and share lots of examples. Becoming familiar with them enables you to:

1. Pinpoint your prevalent style(s) of table talk and decipher unintended messages it may convey.

2. Observe the actual (as opposed to hoped-for) impact of certain table talk on both you and your child.

3. Recognize that you can intentionally change your table talk.

Taken together, these insights get you moving in a new direction and give you access to a better lever for helping your kids while they eat. The objective in this chapter is not to change your language (yet) but to get familiar with common types of table talk, so you can classify your own words and explore their impact on both you and your kids. This can help you feel less powerless at mealtime.

The Power of Words

Transforming your table talk gives you a new kind of nimbleness when parenting around food, which really helps since it's hard to get kids to eat well. A child's distraction (or stalling) at dinner activates our desire to govern the situation. The untouched salad triggers thoughts about the terrible way they've been eating lately, and we catastrophize. Even when we successfully manage our emotions, uncertainty often remains about what to say to elicit the desired outcome. In my case, it was how could I get my kid to eat that salad?

My words, "Eat some salad so you'll be strong for gymnastics," seemed relevant. Healthy eating does, in fact, correlate with improved athletic performance, but this type of table talk did nothing to connect with my daughter or inspire her to eat. In the end, curiosity phrased as an open-ended question, is what worked.

My invitation to explore touch—specifically eat salad with our hands—broke the spell. "I wonder what happens when you crush a crouton?" I asked, watching her eyes light up. This open-ended table talk question got us cracking croutons in half, marveling at their crispness. Quickly, and of her own accord, my daughter began "making presents." She wrapped crouton fragments in salad leaves, then dipped them in dressing. She ate all her salad, then asked for more.

The simple table talk technique of asking an open-ended question launched our unconventional salad, savored part and parcel by hand. I consider this a win, not only because it was conflict-free but because my daughter was wholly engaged as an eater. She was eager, inquisitive, and eating not because I said so but because she was genuinely curious. The Table Talk Method is about that dual shift—of words and mindset—embracing curiosity and replacing exasperation with exploration.

You'll get an entire collection of new table talk later in the book, and as tempting as it may be to skip ahead for quick answers, I encourage you to do the work of every chapter in turn. The material builds upon itself, and completing each section cumulatively supports your longevity and success with the Table Talk Method. Going step-by-step will give you all the tools you need and the depth of understanding to keep things going on your own.

Old Table Talk Traps

In *Child of Mine*, social worker and registered dietitian Ellyn Satter, says: "Family meals are spoiled as parents plead, threaten, bribe, and short-order cook to get children to eat. These practices are so contrary to effective feeding that I'm not entirely sure why they persist" (2000, 31). I'm not sure, either, but I do know how easy it is to fall into these traps, say, at the end of a long day when tempers are short and everyone's hangry or boiling over at dinner.

Parents don't mean to miss the mark when serving up table talk. We've never been trained what to say! More than that, words uttered during meals usually aren't weighed in advance. They fly off our tongue but are below our radar in terms of anticipating effects. Besides, feeding kids is a fickle process! Even with just the right food, served precisely when hunger strikes, we often find ourselves in turmoil at the table.

By the end of this chapter you'll answer these three questions:

1. What's your dominant type of table talk?

2. How does your table talk affect your child's eating behavior?

3. What results do you get with these words?

Getting to the bottom of this begins by examining eight ways things usually go wrong.

Eight Types of Table Talk Unmasked

Over the years I've classified common table talk into eight types: instructive, corrective, praise, conditional, obligatory, expectant, and appreciative table talk and closed-ended questions. I created this framework to teach parents about table talk and help them get a better grip on what they might want to change. This chapter is a deep dive in to each type of table talk, but here's a quick preview of what's coming.

Instructive table talk tells your child what to do or eat. Corrective table talk tries to fix a perceived problem with how or what they're eating (or avoiding). Praise table talk compliments kids' eating, which is different from appreciative table talk, which thanks them for things like good manners or adequate vegetable intake. Conditional table talk gives or withholds food (or rewards) in exchange for eating something else or doing a certain task. Obligatory table talk mandates trying or not wasting food, and expectant table talk tells a kid how they should feel about what they're eating. Finally, closed-ended questions, which prompt dead-end answers like "Yes" or "No," make up an entire category of table talk because they're the polar opposite of what we want.

In the descriptions that follow, "What parents say" lists real-life examples from my research. "What kids hear" shares how kids might interpret and misconstrue those words. I'll then give a brief overview of the unhelpful elements in that genre of table talk. What you're about to read is not meant to make you feel like you're making mistakes. Don't equate familiarity with these words as a sign of failure or reason to denigrate yourself. It's simply a chance to recognize the times and places where a new approach might help. Chapters 6 through 8 cover how to replace these words with new table talk.

1. Instructive Table Talk

Instructive table talk is classic command language. Parents telling kids precisely how and what to do as they eat.

What parents say: "Try this. You might like it."

"Lean over your plate, please."

"Chew with your mouth closed."

"Have another bite."

"Just hold your nose and take a drink afterward."

"Use your napkin."

"Sit down." "Slow down." "Hurry up."

"Please be a good eater."

"Focus on eating."

"Finish your dinner; it's getting cold."

"Just leave it on the side of your plate."

What kids hear: "You've got a lot to learn about eating, so I'll tell you how to do it (by repeating myself again and again). Eat how I say."

Instructive table talk ranges from gentle tutelage to brazen drill-sergeant style. It's specific directions spoken at kids in the act of eating, meant to guide their form and conduct in accomplishing the task. A certain amount of instructive table talk is unavoidable in kids' early years, but its effectiveness declines sharply when they reach preschool age. When assessing table talk tendencies, many parents find instructive table talk festering in situations where its utility has long since elapsed. Parents must teach kids food etiquette in a developmentally appropriate manner, but instructive table talk makes that process hard on everyone.

2. Corrective Table Talk

Corrective table talk implies a child is doing something wrong or different from what parents expect in that moment of eating.

What parents say: "Stop eating with your hands."

"Don't chew with your mouth open."

"Not such big bites!"

"We don't wander around the room eating."

"Quit playing with your food!"

"Don't wipe your face on your sleeve!"

"That's enough mac and cheese. You need to eat some broccoli."

What kids hear: "No! You're doing it all wrong. You're bad at eating. (You are bad.)"

Eating is, by nature, a highly personal act. That means it's difficult for kids to separate commentary about their eating behavior from thoughts and feelings about their character and personhood. Corrective table talk is not intended to be harmful or counterproductive, of course; it's meant to assist in establishing a certain level of proficiency and finesse around eating. The problem is, signaling kids' shortcomings with repetitive messages about what they're doing wrong rarely results in meaningful behavior change. It's anybody's guess, at any given moment, if a child will dismiss, ignore, or imprint corrective table talk. Less uncertain, however, is the redundant nature of these cues and their relative ineffectiveness.

Again, etiquette isn't off-limits, but how social graces are taught is worth reconsidering. A certain measure of parenting success seems hitched to the ability to produce good-natured, well-rounded eaters capable of sitting still and eating varietally. I think that's malarkey, but it's a big reason parents use corrective table talk, which doesn't usually end up helping them achieve that goal anyway. It just grates on both kids' and parents' nerves.

3. Praise Table Talk

Praise table talk is parents commending things they like about a child's eating.

What parents say: "Good job with dinner tonight!"

"I like how you're trying new things!"

"Nice job eating your vegetables."

"What a good eater!"

"I'm impressed you sat and ate all of your dinner!"

"Great job finishing!"

What kids hear: "Eating well (or according to the rules) makes you good and worthy."

Wanting to compliment a job well done is natural, especially if eating is a challenge with your child. The problem with praise is it thrusts parental approval into the mix of things kids must sort out as eaters. Kids unfailingly aim to please their parents. This means when self-discovery and autonomy of eating get mixed up with wanting accolades, kids might eat for the wrong reasons. Praise isn't meant to induce internal conflict, but it causes kids to juggle extrinsic factors (like pleasing their parents) with trying to explore food and their eating.

4. Conditional Table Talk

Conditional table talk is if-you-eat-this-you-can-have-that type talk. It makes eating dependent on some other circumstance(s), including food, behavior, or other activities or events.

What parents say: "You need to finish your veggies if you want dessert."

"Eat two more bites of chicken; then you can have more pasta."

"If you use your fingers, I'm taking it away."

"Goofing around at dinner means no TV time later."

"If you want to have energy to play, you need to eat a healthy meal."

"Just try some. If you don't like it, you can have something else."

"If your room is clean before soccer, we can get ice cream on the way home."

What kids hear: "If you eat this or do this…then you earn something better." Or, inversely, "If you don't eat this or do this…then you don't deserve the thing you really want."

Conditional table talk is the opening act in a circuitous play, where food is one of two diametric things: worthy, delicious, and desirable or two-bit, dull, and required. The food-as-reward-or-punishment trap is as old as eating itself, and while no parent intends to perpetuate this system, conditional table talk persists, fueling these familiar axioms:

- If you eat the unpleasant stuff, then you deserve a reward (food or otherwise).

- If you don't eat the necessary stuff, you earn a penalty (food or otherwise).

- If you do a good job or succeed, you deserve a food-based reward.

- If you fail or fall short, you deserve a food-based punishment.

Conditional table talk sets up a dicey rubric of eating that can snowball over a lifetime. The unintended outcome of conditional table talk is that kids grow up learning to reward and punish themselves using food. This conundrum is a source of guilt and shame many adults want help undoing. A bad day at work begets a pint of ice cream, and stomaching salad "justifies the cheeseburger." Decoupling food and behavior is a critical skill parents can teach with new table talk.

Similarly, bribing kids to take two more bites so they can get something better (that is, dessert) doesn't promote healthy eating. It teaches kids to bypass inner cues to get "superior" food or their parent's approval. The same goes for wielding food-related promises or guarantees (about health or incentives, like a new video game). Food should not be dependent on (or withheld) because of how kids act or eat.

5. Obligatory Table Talk

Obligatory table talk imposes compulsory eating, saying you must at least give food(s) a try. This type of table talk comes in three varieties: necessity, scarcity, and liability. Each sub-type is must-do, have-to, arm-twisting lingo that mandates eating based on several factors, many of which are fact-based but just not particularly motivating from a kid's point of view. The crown jewel of obligatory table talk is the *try-bite* rule (also called the *one-bite* rule or *no-thank-you bite*). We'll explore this in depth below.

VARIETY 1: NECESSITY

This is the garden-variety form of obligatory table talk, issuing a basic mandate or "you must" phrase around food.

What parents say: "Try this; it's good for you."

"You have to try at least one bite."

"Just try it again; you might like it this time."

"You need to try it before you decide you don't like it." ("Twenty-nine more chances!")

"You don't have to like it, but you do have to try it."

"Okay. Well, show me trying."

What kids hear: "You don't know enough to be trusted to decide about trying this food. I know what's best for you. Eat it anyway. I'll hound you until you put some in your mouth. Then (maybe) you can tell me how you feel."

Obligatory table talk's best-known tactic—the try-bite—is usually invoked when kids don't want to eat a certain food. This tactic aspires to make kids feel entitled to their opinion ("Try some. You might like it!"), but fails paradoxically because it robs them of any real right to choose. This type of language isn't unique to eating. It comes up at other times when parents compel kids to do stuff they'd rather skip, like cleaning their room. Whining and procrastination can ensue, no matter how simple the task. Eventually kids must pick up the toys and socks whether they want to or not. So parents feel justified saying "You don't have to like it. You just need to do it!" Maybe this works for chores, but it's fishy when applied to eating, because eating well is different from mastering other life skills (see chapter 1).

The biggest problems with obligatory table talk are how it squelches curiosity and how it eliminates agency around eating. But dropping this type of table talk can be hard, for any number of reasons:

- Some parents believe their child won't try new foods unless mandated.

- They presume these forced occasion tries will eventually lead their child to feel favorable toward or at least tolerate that food.

- They think obligatory table talk empowers kids, especially if their version of the try-bite includes the "freedom" to dislike it.

- It's a deeply familiar type of table talk, reminiscent of language they themselves heard during childhood.

These are a few of the reasons why transforming table talk involves changing your words and your mindset.

One thing is clear about obligatory table talk: kids who are forced to try food, even when "permitted" to dislike it, remember less about the food and more about how they felt being required to eat it. Not surprisingly, they don't usually like the food (by association or otherwise). Asking a child to taste something while saying they don't have to like it pushes three undesirable agendas:

1. Kids learn to be less reliant on internal cues around food desires, hunger, and satiety.

2. Kids feel bamboozled, being told they can offer an opinion about food but not decide (and share details about) whether or not they feel like eating it.

3. Kids dig in their heels to demonstrate independence as an eater.

Many of my adult clients share stories about childhood battles over food that left them with a longstanding distaste for certain foods.

VARIETY 2 : SCARCITY

Scarcity table talk goes down the path of *others have less than you*. It often comes from the intention to teach kids about privilege and the preciousness of food along with helping them recognize the value of not wasting food. Unfortunately, the words often said are a throwback to clean-plate club banter that turns shame and guilt into stimuli for eating.

What parents say: "You're lucky to have oatmeal for breakfast! Many kids wish they had this food."

"Some kids are going to bed with no food tonight, so please eat your dinner."

"You took it, so you're going to have to eat it."

"Mush it up all you want, but you're not going to waste that."

What kids hear: "Shame on you for not doing a better job eating."

Food insecurity (globally as well as in the United States) is an incredibly serious problem. According to Feeding America (2018), one in six American children goes hungry on a regular basis (this was prior to the Covid-19 pandemic). That's irrefutably atrocious in this "land of plenty," and more must be done to end childhood hunger. That said, it's best for parents to avoid table talk that presumes kids will eat well out of deference to peers, known or unknown, experiencing the torment of insufficient food. As your child comes of age, you can talk with them and get involved in activism against hunger, but bringing these things up as a way to get your kids eating better leads nowhere good.

Urging a child to eat oatmeal because they are fortunate enough to possess it dispenses pressure undercut with judgment. An innuendo of shame, like "What's the matter with you? You ought to be gobbling this up!" can bring about adverse associations. Stable access to food is something to be grateful for, but it's dangerous fodder for spurring kids to eat, because it links feeling bad, about themselves or situations, as a precursor to eating.

Imagine using the equivalent of scarcity table talk with your child about a book they didn't want to read. It would sound something like this: "You're lucky to have this book! Just look at all these chapters—and this exhilarating plot! There are a lot of kids in the world who wish they could read this." This sounds off-the-wall when talking about reading, but it rolls off the tongue when it comes to eating.

VARIETY 3: LIABILITY

The liability version of obligatory table talk imposes external pressure on kids to eat because of the effort or sacrifice of someone or something else.

What parents say:	"Food costs money, you know."
	"We work hard to buy good food. Please don't waste it."
	"The earth grew this food for us."
	"I spent a lot of time making this, so I would appreciate it if you would at least try it."
What kids hear:	"Eating is duty bound. You're on the hook to eat because people (and the environment) work hard to make it happen. Eat to avoid disgrace."
They also may hear	"You are ungrateful."
	"You owe it to me."
	"I did this for you. Now return the favor. Eat this for me."

Food is undeniably expensive, effortful, and precious, yet coaxing kids to eat from this perspective rarely induces gratitude. Asking kids to eat out of indebtedness can stir up a sense of stress and dishonor. These matters of eating can contribute to heart-wrenching beliefs. Gloria, a longtime client of mine, once said of her childhood relationship to food, "I was trained to 'waist it' rather than waste it."

6. Expectant Table Talk

Expectant table talk imposes a parent's opinion of how the child will (or should) feel about a food or eating experience, telling them what to expect or experience while eating.

What parents say:	"I made it just how you like!"
	"This is delicious! I think you're really going to like it!"
	"Your food will get cold, and it won't taste very good."
	"You loved this last time we had it?!"
	"The crust is the best part!"
	"You must not be very hungry right now."
	"You're almost done!"
	"It's just chicken, which you eat all the time."
	"This tastes just like X, and you like that."
	"If you try it a bunch, you get used to new flavors."
	"This is so yummy! I wouldn't feed you something that tastes bad."
What kids hear:	"You should have this experience. What you like or don't like is less reliable than my knowledge, opinions, or recollections of your likes and dislikes."

These words of pseudo encouragement don't help kids eat better. "I think this food is amazing, and therefore you should too" is not an argument that triggers a kid's interest in eating. In fact, it usually awakens their inner contrarian. Skittish and skeptical culinary connoisseurs, children want to eat on their own terms. Associations, determinations, and understandings about food are for kids to forge, not for parents to project.

The same goes for reminding kids they liked a food the last time they tried it. Since eating always happens in the present moment, it's not helpful to persuade kids to do anything with food based on what happened before. Last time, they might have eaten it just to get a parent off their back! Even when a kid isn't totally averse to a food, being told how they should feel eating it can cause bitterness that overshadows everything else. Encouraging kids to eat from a "See, I told you so!" perspective doesn't help them like new foods or believe in themselves as eaters.

7. Appreciative Table Talk

Appreciative table talk means thanking your child for an eating job well done.

What parents say:	"Thanks for trying."
	"Thank you for at least tasting it!"
	"Thanks for using such good manners."
What kids hear:	"When you eat properly, it pleases me."
	This suggests that parental contentedness is relevant and valuable when it comes to kids' eating.

Appreciative table talk is an overt expression of gratitude for some aspect of kids' eating, and it's enticing due to its Pavlovian potential. Parents want to laud their child's on-point efforts at the table, and they hope this kind of table talk will reinforce desired behaviors. At first glance, most parents wonder, what's wrong with appreciative table talk?

By now you won't be surprised to hear that appreciating a child for eating well can send an undesirable message. With appreciative table talk, a kid's recognition of their self-worth as an eater becomes tied to opinions and judgments parents offer about how they're performing around food. The obvious complexity is that parents have a role in helping kids eat, but appreciating their efforts with stand-alone thank-yous is a missed opportunity to nurture their self-efficacy. The key to transforming appreciative table talk is to ask kids an open-ended question in place of blanket words of appreciation, something you'll learn to practice in chapter 7.

8. Closed-Ended Questions

Table talk in the form of a closed-ended question is phrasing your question in a way that prompts a very short, often one-word answer like "Yes," "No," or "Because."

What parents say:	"Do you like the carrots?"
	"Did you taste the potatoes?"
	"Are you going to try the peas?"
	"Can you tell me why you don't like it?"
	"Remember how hungry you are when you don't eat dinner?"
What kids hear:	Nagging or badgering in the form of "I may be asking you for thoughts or feelings about food, but the agenda is getting you to eat."

A central theme in my table talk research is that parents rarely use table talk phrased as a question, and when table talk is in the form of a question, it's usually unhelpful (closed-ended). Closed-ended questions constrict parents' efforts to promote healthy eating (more on this in chapter 6). They're a category of table talk unto themselves for a couple of reasons. First, they are the most common table talk mistake. Moreover, parents who adjust this type of table talk report fewer food struggles with their kids even when it's the only thing they adjust.

Hearing about all eight types of table talk can be dizzying. It's not easy to accept what might come from old table talk, especially if it sounds all too familiar. Rest assured that this is a normal reaction. And in my experience, it doesn't last. But it's good to remember that feeling bad about yourself, your table talk, or what it's doing to your child will not yield better results. You are good enough. You are doing great work, and you're turning the tables on how you relate to your child over food. With that in mind, the next step is to examine your table talk tendencies.

What Do You Make of Your Words?

All eight kinds of table talk arise from earnest intentions, yet they routinely sabotage parents' efforts at getting kids eating well. The impact of typical table talk can be summarized in three universal themes:

1. It doesn't get kids eating more or better.

2. It's rife with redundancy. Parents keep saying the same things and landing in the same spot.

3. It leaves both parents and kids feeling disempowered.

Understanding your table talk tendencies gives you the option to break free of those words and to move on to more meaningful and effective communication with your kids over food. The next exercise is a simple matching task to identify your typical table talk styles.

EXERCISE: Your Table Talk Audit

Turn to the list of table talk quotes you've collected in your journal so far. Use the chart below to compare your words to the examples from this chapter. Where do your words match up? Which examples sound most like the table talk on your own list? These are your dominant types of table talk. Note them in your journal.

Eight Types of Table Talk

Table Talk Type	Message	Example Quote
Instructive	*Do this.*	"Please use your fork."
Corrective	*Not that.*	"Stop using your hands." "Don't talk with your mouth full."
Praise	*Good job! I'm so proud of you!*	"Way to go eating your vegetables!"
Conditional	*If you do X, then Y will be possible.*	"Eat two more bites, then you can..."
Obligatory	*You have to eat.*	"Just try one bite." "Don't waste that!" "I worked hard making this. Please eat some."
Expectant	*This is how or what you should feel.* *This is how you could feel if you tried!* *This is how you've felt before.*	"This tastes just like X, which you like!" "I think you're going to love it!"
Appreciative	*I'm grateful for how you are eating.*	"Thank you for tasting it!"
Closed-ended questions	*There's a simple yes or no response.*	"Did you try the soup?" "Are you going to drink your milk?"

Most parents use two or three main types of table talk. Others use a smattering of this and that, depending on the situation. There's no point comparing how many categories you use (or what you use) with what other adults in your life do, because no single kind of table talk is worse than another. Please don't conclude you're doing a terrible job even if you recognize your own voice in every single type listed. This process is simply meant to help you identify and understand your usual table talk, so you can step back and begin to transform it.

Once you've identified your main types of table talk, your task is noticing what these words do. With your journal in hand, over the next few days, pay close attention to how your child responds to your table talk. What do they do, eat, or say in reaction to your words? Watch and listen closely, and then write down what you observe using the following instructions.

Self-Reflection Journaling

At the top of a clean page in your journal write "Table Talk Effects." Over the next three days, keep track of what you observe happening in relation to your table talk. This includes how your child interacts with you over food in addition to what they eat or resist eating and how they behave during meals and snacks. You want raw data from your own table, so write down whatever you hear and see. The quickest way to do this is to answer these prompts in your journal:

- *My child replies to my typical table talk by saying*:

- *My child responds to my typical table talk by doing*:

- *Using typical table talk makes me feel*:

At the end of three days, review what you've written down. How do these results compare to what you want? Don't try to change your table talk yet, but just watch for correlations. Connect the dots between what you say and how your child responds, both in words and behaviors. Remember that investigating your table talk can feel enlightening and daunting. Turn up the volume of self-awareness without getting caught up in self-judgment. If this is feeling difficult, reread the section at the end of chapter 2 on how to stop judging yourself (and others) for table talk.

With your table talk audit complete, you've reached a defining moment. Your current language is on the docket for change, so we need to differentiate between what you've said all along and the new and improved stuff you're going to adopt. To accomplish this, we'll start referring to table talk as either *old* or *new*. The unhelpful stuff you're trying to change, then, is old table talk (all the examples in chapter 3). The more desirable language you learn from here on out will be new table talk. For the rest of the book, you'll be moving from old to new table talk.

With lingo sorted, you're ready to lay a new foundation, because new words work best when their origins are clear. The bedrock of new table talk is curiosity and connection, which is what we'll explore next.

CHAPTER 4

Meet the Eater, Your Child

Six-month-old Suri is on the verge of starting solids. She is fascinated with food despite never having taken one bite. Fixing her gaze on the eaters around her, she opens and closes her tiny lips, chewing air. And so, it begins. Precious mimicry launching the lifelong adventure of learning about oneself as an eater.

This moment in time is unique for both Suri and her parents. Every food she encounters is brand new. Suri's gung ho! Seeing, smelling, touching, tongue thrusting, and two-fisting baby spoons that are more like catapults, percussion instruments, and gag inducers than utensils. Every morsel of table food is an adventure for Suri. And this is all happening in a relative table talk void.

Suri is observing external cues and striving to assimilate. She's relating what she witnesses about eating to her sensory-rich internal experience. Attuning to this inner world involves connecting with experienced eaters in her presence, then exploring and aligning her behaviors with what she sees and hears from them. And what they offer is heartfelt affirmation and encouragement. The people she loves and trusts cheer her on most attentively. It's a momentous unfolding.

What if future grown-up Suri could know this likeness of herself as an eater? The built-in curiosity and connectedness she relies on as she relates to food are core elements of eating invaluable for her to retain. Suri deserves and depends on certain latitudes and gratifications while eating, which she gets in droves from both her parents and food.

Suri is months, if not years, away from full-fledged meltdowns over food. And her parents have very specific ways of relating to her as she eats. They're using skills and behaviors rooted in curiosity and connectivity that flow almost automatically between parents and kids at this age. When I say curiosity, I mean a genuine interest that leads to a question. And by connection (or connectedness), I mean joining together to feel a sense of partnership.

If you currently have a baby just starting solid food, you're living the material in this chapter. For the rest of us, well, the shine is probably off. But it's never too late to recapture how you keep kids in the game with food. Curiosity and connection help you improve eating interactions whether you're feeding toddlers or teens. It's not a lost cause if food freak-outs happen daily (or at every meal) in your home. Meaningful change comes from understanding how to bring curiosity and connection back to both your words and actions while eating with kids. To make this less nebulous, let's turn back the clock to a time when eating-related challenges weren't so pervasive. Hidden there are useful clues to solve your food struggles today.

Rewinding the Clock

Looking back reminds you of what kids need to thrive as eaters: curiosity and connection with food. Your job as a parent is to recognize and nurture these core elements of eating so they endure beyond the high chair. For this to work, you need engaging ways to sustain kids' penchant for eating. But what are those skills? And how do you strengthen them, especially if you're stuck in unrelenting food battles?

One way to identify what you can do is through comparing your interactions with your kid over food today with your interactions of yesteryear. What has changed about how you relate to your child as they eat? How are you engaging around food today versus what's in the rearview mirror?

The next exercise takes you on a trip down memory lane to explore two things: what your child was like as an eater early on and how your parenting around food has changed since then. It's a personalized exploration of differences you'd probably expect to see between Suri eating at six months compared to, say, her eating at the age of six. The less conscious part is how much parenting practices shift in a relatively short span of time.

EXERCISE: Meet-Your-Eater Quiz and Reflections

Scroll through your phone archives or a photo album for a video or an image of your child eating in the first year or two of their life. If your child is younger than two, find a picture of them eating from as far back as you can. It doesn't matter what, where, or how they're eating. If you can't find a picture of your own child eating, use the "Baby Eating a Banana" video link available at http://www.newharbinger.com/49463.

Write "Meet the Eater" at the top of a new page in your journal. Now study the photo or watch the video, and then answer the following questions. Write your responses down instead of keeping them in your head. Brief comments are all you need. Base your answers on what you see and feel from the picture or from the video alone (this part of the exercise is *not about your eating concerns today*).

1. What is your child using to eat? Include body parts and utensils as specifically as you can. Fingers, hands, fists, a fork, spoon, spatula, chopsticks, or anything else?

2. Where is their food besides in their mouth? Is it on their lips, cheeks, chin, nose, forehead, eyes, brows, hands, or hair? How about on their shirt and the floor? Record everything that applies.

3. What words best describe how your child is relating to their food? How exploratory is your child as they eat in this situation?

4. Which of the five senses do you imagine are engaged? Sight, smell, touch, taste, sound? List all that apply.

5. What's your child's mood in this photo or video?

Now imagine traveling back in time and sitting face-to-face with your child in this moment of eating. Put yourself into the picture. Nostalgia aside, what feelings come up for you?

6. Describe the energy and attention you used in this moment of eating. What did it take? What kind of effort and presence were happening on your end?

7. How were you honoring your child as an eater? What was your primary focus? What was your main struggle (besides cleaning up)?

8. Based on your reflections, what would you say is at the heart of who your child is as an eater?

There are no right or wrong answers on this quiz. These are personal observations meant to help you call to mind the wisdom you already possess. To do that, turn to the next page in your journal and use your answers from questions 3, 4, and 5 to respond to this set of writing prompts:

- What about your child's eating is the same today as the baby you fed back then? Not mechanics or messiness, but who's showing up at the table? What matters to them?

- How is your child still curious about eating today even amidst their headstrong habits?

- What skills did you previously use to care for your child's limited experience as an eater?

Your insights offer a glimpse into your child's essence as an eater today. These qualities still want to thrive, and you can learn how to feed that.

Now read your answers to questions 6 and 7 from the quiz and use them to respond to these writing prompts:

- Which of the things that you identified are still going strong today in food interactions with your child?

- How does your attention and energy during meals today differ from how it used to be? Rather than judging it as "better" or "worse," list specific behaviors or attitudes that have changed in how you interact with your child as they eat.

· What's your focus in feeding your child today? What's your top priority in terms of their eating?

Kids need time to evolve as eaters, but how we parent them around food changes fast. In the first few years, we lean in with patience, playfulness, and permissiveness. We handle emotions and inefficiencies with tolerance and tenderness, and a certain kind of sweetness abounds despite the annoying bits. Food literally crusts on our walls, floor, and clothes, exhausting our aching backs, but somehow our sense of joy and possibility remains intact. The parental moxie you used to create that kind of eating environment with your kid is waiting in the wings.

Feeding kids of any age can be messy and demanding work, with aggravation, gratification, and everything in between. There's no silver bullet to eliminate worry about how and what kids eat, but you can consciously recognize that your fears and frustrations don't constitute the whole story. You can also revive competencies and goodwill, which you already possess, and strengthen skills of curiosity and connection. Doing this is imperative for helping kids eat well.

Curiosity and Connection

In the earliest months and years of eating, we're present with kids in unique ways. We sit with them face-to-face or maybe even welcome them onto our lap, offering an intimate eating experience. We catch their eyes and attune to their smiles and grimaces with genuine intrigue. We're absorbed and entertained by their facial contortions when new textures and flavors are explored. Feeding them is demanding and auspicious, but we show up in a grounded way, steeped in present-moment attentiveness and imperturbability.

We cut, mash, and moisten foods, expecting amounts eaten will be small. We open wide to fistfuls of food yo-yoing in and out of our child's mouth and retrieve slobbery utensils flung through the air repeatedly. We stand guard for the grand finale (aka smash-n-smear); sometimes we laugh, other times we snap, but we aren't surprised that it happens. A good portion of foods we serve never even make it to our kid's stomach. And we accept that. Just like we do when their bowl of soup gets impulsively worn as a hat. Noodles and broth dripping off your head is either exhilarating or exasperating, depending on whether you are a child or their parent. This series of events, behaviors, and meager intake isn't labeled a meltdown when kids are very young. When does that change, and how do we get there in the span of just a few years?

A friend told me about her two-year-old son's latest eating trick. He ends each meal by quickly shoving as much food as he can into his ears. He finds it hilarious, while his parents now face an unexpected challenge: serving foods small enough not to lodge in his esophagus but large enough to avoid being crammed in his ear. When parenting infants and toddlers around food, we view shenanigans as part of the process. We embolden all kinds of exploration with food and the act of eating itself. Investigating smell, sound, touch, texture, and mouth feel of food are sanctioned activities approached with utmost curiosity by babies and parents alike!

When kids are very young eaters, we are optimally engaged. We're authentically interested and openly inquisitive during moments of eating together. We mimic chewing and make throaty sounds like "Mmmm" and "Nom-nom-nom." We say, "How is that?" or "Is it tasting yummy?!" The fact that we ask babies—without the ability to reply in words yet—questions about their direct experience of eating shows that our basic inclination when feeding kids is one of symbiotic curiosity.

Remember when you used to mime acts of eating for your child? Exaggerating chomping with your mouth, tongue, and teeth, then embellishing those maneuvers with nonverbal antics and guttural noises never used before or since. Those moments are part of the fabric connecting you and your child around eating, and regardless of your feeding struggles today, those threads remain unbroken. The answer is not regressing to spoon feeding or flying-food-airplane games but actively rekindling curiosity and connectedness in developmentally up-leveled ways.

We listen to and trust babies with their experiences of eating in ways we tend to forget later. Take baby sign language, for example. This is when parents teach infants to communicate things about eating like "more" and "all done" using hand and finger gestures. Babies know how to consult their inner barometer of eating and pantomime what they want and need with food long before they can tell us with words. As parents, we rely on their know-how to maintain harmony during meals. We trust their awareness and ability to let us know what's going on for them as eaters. This is the kind of interaction we need to rekindle with our kids while they eat today.

Five things we reliably offer kids in their earliest years of eating:

1. Our attentive presence while they eat

2. Freedom to explore without a requirement to eat

3. Verbalized interest in their food and eating experience

4. Patience for both playfulness and "contrary" behavior

5. Belief in their inner wisdom and ability to find their way with food

How prominent are these things when eating with your child today?

What We Lost Along the Way

As parents we embrace a depth of curiosity in the earliest phase of our kid's eating, and then somehow lose track of that instinct. We intentionally foster wonderment around eating for a short period of time relative to how long it takes to grow the life skill of eating well. Somewhere around toddlerhood, we start treating kids differently while they eat. They've got the logistics, so we shift gears and begin prioritizing things like "variety" and "balanced intake." With this comes more knowingness and less patience during meals, on the part of both parents and kids.

Developmental benchmarks focus on kids mastering the fine motor skills of eating. As soon as they safely and reliably ingest food independently, they start to lose parents' active encouragement to eat in an exploratory and interconnected way. Sadly, that means we lose touch with the most mindful elements of eating when kids are very young. The change isn't detectable day by day, but in the span of a few short years, we drop the curious and connected qualities we used to bring to the table.

As kids grow up, we grow away from certain ways of relating to them as they eat, to the point where we think kids are "becoming pickier" or "less enthusiastic about healthy food" when, in fact, how we interact with them around food and eating is probably the bigger culprit. This happens with kids from preschool on up and includes things said about their eating when we're not even there for the meal. I mean comments made when your grade-schooler's lunch box comes home largely untouched or when your high-schooler orders Uber Eats to your basement from their phone. How do you talk with your kid about that? Maybe it's not happening (yet). But what do you imagine saying? Do those words originate from curiosity and connection?

Over time, rules, social norms, and expectations get applied to kids as they eat, conditioning out curiosity and dampening connectedness over food. This usually happens by way of old table talk. Things we say to kids about eating infuse a low-grade pressure, blanketing their eating experiences with a kind of humdrum effect. Without even realizing it, we wind up promoting kids' disengagement with food. Meltdowns begin, old table talk mushrooms, and before we know it, we're caught in a vicious cycle. But it doesn't have to stay this way. Curiosity and connectedness are powerful antidotes to impasses over food with your kids.

Whatever food quandary you face today, trust that it will change. Three, five, or ten years from now, what bothers you about your child's eating won't be the same. That's the nature of feeding kids. And the nature of being a parent. Two habitudes you embraced feeding your child early on in life are curiosity and connection, and these are things you can consistently rely on to deal with food conflict. The new table talk and parenting practices you'll learn next help you bring this spirit back to your table.

New Table Talk

Your new table talk begins with two sentence stems to reestablish curiosity and connection. Their purpose is to convey an interest in exploration and a sense of partnership. Start using these two new phrases as often as you can during meals: "What do you notice…" and "Tell me about…"

This new table talk can be used anytime, but I recommend trying it when your child complains about a food. Sniveling about squash means you ask, "What do you notice about the squash?" When kids reply, "It's mushy and gross," say, "Tell me about the gross part for you." Then listen actively. Make space for your child to share freely without making them eat squash.

Start using these new phrases daily, remembering their purpose is to awaken curiosity and connection. You're not using new table talk to make your kids eat stuff. You're demonstrating that what they notice about food is something worth caring about and that eating in your home is you-plus-me instead of you-versus-me. These are big steps toward undoing old patterns that fuel mealtime angst.

Use your new table talk phrases when things go poorly and also when they go well. When your child delights in a food, no matter how healthy or unhealthy you deem it to be, ask "What do you notice…" or "Tell me about…" so your table talk becomes "What do you notice about cheese puffs?" or "Tell me about the ice cream." This new table talk shows your child that their experience of food really matters, not in terms of dictating what's for dinner but in terms of learning to drop in and notice eating as it's happening.

My friend Libby is a nutritionist and mom of three teens, ages nineteen, sixteen, and thirteen. Her youngest has a hankering for convenience store snacks and the money and means to get them. She's torn because he eats homecooked meals full of colorful garden-grown plants but also grabs Doritos and Milk Duds as a predinner snack. Rather than try to convince him not to buy or eat these foods, I suggested Libby ask him what he loves most about Doritos and Milk Duds.

It might make you nervous you're giving the green light when you say, "Tell me about Doritos for you," but that's the difference between old and new table talk. Old table talk comes from a place of fear, worry, frustration, judgment, or disbelief. It extols balanced intake, regulation, variety, and all kinds of nutrition stuff you can count, like protein, carbs, vitamins, or how much kids eat. New table talk isn't like that. It's asked from a place of curiosity and connection, and it aims to nurture gastro-nomic intelligence (we'll cover that in chapter 5).

The quiz you took at the start of this chapter was a reminder of your child's basic aptitude and vitality as an eater. It took you back to a time when you prioritized their process of eating over rating how or what they ate. You can't revert to feeding kids like you did when they were a baby, but you must reignite those skills of curiosity and connectedness in intentional and relevant ways. New table talk does this for you, freeing you and your child from fixed ideas about food and who they are as an eater, someone who is not "picky" but just right. New table talk helps you find the sweet spot of relating to your child as they eat, which makes conflict less likely no matter what's for dinner.

Implementing new table talk rooted in curiosity and connection might sound like idealistic fluff, but it reduces struggles over food in two tangible ways. It improves how you relate to your child while they eat (creating less friction) and it invigorates the relationship between your child and their food (captivating appeal). But curiosity and connection don't just happen with words. Certain action steps will elevate their presence during meals. Six such practices are outlined in the next section.

Six Ways to Revitalize Curiosity and Connection

The behaviors below are practical ways to reinvigorate curiosity and connection while eating with your child. These practices work with new table talk to diffuse mealtime stress and remind you to meet your eater where they're at.

1. Keep all tech off the table when you eat with your child. Putting your smartphone facedown beside you won't cut it. Store devices out of view, reach, and earshot for the duration of time you eat with your child. This is vital for establishing true connection. It might be hard to do, but it gives you a leg to stand on when your kid is old enough to have a phone and won't put it down during meals.

2. Be fully present, even if you only have a few minutes. Feel your backside touching your chair, take a mindful breath in, and bring attentiveness of your mind and body to what's happening here with food.

3. Model eating behavior you'd like to see replicated, without broadcasting it. I call this *show-not-tell eating*. In other words, eat your veggies without declaring how great they taste or how healthy they are. If you just can't hold back, say only one adjective followed by a question. Say, "This eggplant is *tangy*." Then ask, "What do you notice?" or "Tell me about the eggplant for you."

4. Start an origin of food conversation inviting your child to be the storyteller. Say, "I wonder where eggplant lives when it's growing up?" Then actively listen. If that's too juvenile, ask, "How many varieties of eggplant can we name?" or "I wonder where eggplants grow best?"

5. Avoid commenting on the volume of food your child eats or leaves behind. If you think they're eating too little or too much, keep it to yourself. Rather than say "You haven't eaten much omelet," use new table talk instead. Ask your child, "What do you notice about the omelet?" or "Tell me about the omelet for you." The same goes when they're devouring tacos to the point you think they might burst. Say, "What do you notice about tacos?" or "Tell me about tacos for you!"

6. Recall the energy and attentiveness you described in question 6 of the meet-your-eater quiz: what it was like when you went back in time and remembered sitting face-to-face with your young child eating. You're not starting from scratch. Even if it feels like a distant memory, you can reengage skills you relied on in the past when your child's eating was *literally a mess*. This durability is yours to reclaim, so when your child rejects food, you no longer take it personally or assign greater meaning than is due. When things fall apart over food, remember the picture you found for the meet-your-eater quiz. At their core, that worthy kid is the same person you're feeding today.

With specific ideas for enhancing curiosity and connection, it's time to decide which practices you'll use. Your next journal entry will help you craft a plan to bring curiosity and connection back to eating interactions with your child.

Self-Reflection Journaling

Turn to a clean page in your journal and write "Curiosity and Connection" at the top. Review the six ways to revitalize curiosity and connection, and then answer the next set of questions to decide which action steps you'll take to practice connection and curiosity with your child while you eat.

- Which of these six practices don't happen regularly while eating in your home?

- If you're doing all these things, which ones drop off when food struggles begin?

- Which practices intrigue you (even if you're not sure they'll work)?

- Which could you do every day?

Circle at least one of the ideas you wrote down. If you're scratching your head, pick a practice you suspect your child won't view as babyish. Then try it out regularly when eating with your child. Once you're in a groove with this behavior, add another if you like. Getting all of these practices going eventually helps shore up your new table talk.

Curiosity and connection are prolific when we feed babies; then a downshift in that energy occurs, coinciding with the emergence of old table talk. Reinvigorating curiosity and connection around food is necessary because that's the environment kids need for eating well. In the coming chapters, you'll see how these practices feed a steady stream of new table talk and help kids grow and develop as eaters. One of my clients describes this as "going from trying to get healthy stuff into kids to creating a sense of love, joy, and connection with food." If that's a gap you'd like to close too, the next chapter will show you how.

CHAPTER 5

Nurture Your Family's Gastronomic Intelligence

Curiosity and connection with food come alive through our five senses. For three-year-old Cole, that means a love of peeling clementines. He doesn't eat them yet. Jabbing his thumb through rind after rind, Cole delights in the citrusy release. He strips pithy strands with exquisite care, then piles the orbs up for others to eat. Cole will peel an entire bag of fruit if left unattended, exemplifying how easily kids engage with food on a sensory level.

Exploring touch, smell, sight, and sound of food—even when kids won't eat it— is an important precursor to trying new things and curbing meltdown risk. When it comes to food, where interest goes, engagement follows. When you help kids get curious with food, you up their interest in eating. I mean not just being playful with food but intentionally pinpointing awareness of whatever your senses come into contact with. The smell of sourdough bread baking or the weight of one grape on your tongue. The juicy explosion of biting into a ripe peach in August. This is the stuff driving Cole. No one prods him to lick, taste, or eat clementines, which leaves him free to explore at his own pace, without external pressure. As a result, he has an unencumbered interest in the sight, smell, touch, and succulence of clementines. One day soon, I bet he'll eat a segment not to please anyone other than himself.

Kids' natural inclination is to eat with their full array of senses. Remember the image of your own child from the meet-your-eater quiz in the previous chapter? Kids intuitively fondle, sniff, and squish food from an early age even when they have no intention of eating it. At some point, we deem this wasteful behavior evident of poor table manners. But kids don't care about that. They're truly embodied eaters.

To rekindle curiosity, the next set of skills in the Table Talk Method involves paying attention to your five senses while eating, and practicing this with your kids. It's one of three important ways to nurture gastronomic intelligence. In this chapter you'll learn why GI is vital for raising healthy eaters and decreasing food conflict. You'll also acquire additional new table talk, including a wildly effective phrase for dealing with food rejection issues. Let's begin by coming to our senses.

Tune In to Your Five Senses

Sight, smell, touch, sound, and flavor all play critical roles in how we experience food. I'm talking about being attentive to the sound of a potato chip crunching in your mouth or the tenderness of a vine-ripened raspberry dissolving on your tongue. When was the last time you asked your child about something like that?

Most of the time we eat without paying much attention to the sensations arising in our body and mind with food. Unfortunately, this means we also fail to elicit these observations from our kids. Children naturally eat in a more mindful way, so when we skip over that, we miss the lowest hanging fruit for improving how they eat. Consistently eating with all five senses is an easy way to subvert mealtime struggles and change the dynamics at your family table.

Kids of any age can do this. It doesn't necessitate verbal skills. Observing things like color, smell, temperature, and texture are productive places to begin, because that's already what kids focus on when it comes to food. Think how ravenous your child can be but somehow still take time to rip and smoosh bread into tiny pellets before eating it. Or how they linger to savor every iota of certain foods—it's mind-boggling to watch! Recently, I was devouring chocolate covered pretzels and caught a glimpse of my eight-year-old. Five minutes passed as she methodically licked the first pretzel she'd taken from the bin. Twisting her wrist and maneuvering her tongue, she persisted until every speck of chocolate was gone, one mini pretzel rendered soggy and bare.

Kids eat this way naturally. They're not trying to slow down or get control of themselves or their intake. Nor should they be. They instinctively eat in an inward sort of way, mindfully aware of the moment-to-moment bliss or blech that can come from food. This is an open invitation for us as parents, a way to access more fun and effective feeding methods. Tuning in to your five senses while eating with your child and using language that encourages them do the same is a turning point for ending food conflict, and the curiosity and connection you've revitalized are scaffolding for the process.

Mindful Eating

Bringing awareness to your senses while eating, as I teach it, is one piece of something broadly known as mindful eating. I began studying mindfulness nearly twenty years ago with professional training in mindfulness-based stress reduction as taught by Jon Kabat-Zinn and Saki Santorelli. In the decades since, I have learned from many esteemed teachers including Pema Chödrön, Sharon Salzberg, Tara Brach, Narayan Liebenson, Larry Rosenberg, and Zeenat Potia. I've done research on mindful eating and taught with colleagues from varying backgrounds, all of which I mention because the Table Talk Method has roots in mindfulness. I want to give credit where due.

My ideas have evolved from my personal and professional experiences of mindfulness: the research and the remarkable teachers I've had the good fortune to learn from and with. I practice and teach mindful eating because there's nothing else like it for helping people settle into who they are as eaters. The part of mindful eating I'll share with you here is how to eat with your five senses and teach that to your child in conjunction with new table talk.

What I call *five senses–based eating* means connecting with what's going on in your eyes, ears, nose, mouth, hands, heart, and stomach while you eat. It's awareness of what's happening below your eyebrows:

tuning in to the sight, touch, smell, sound, and flavor of food with present-moment attentiveness to the best of your ability.

When your eyes see a plate of sweet potato fries, what do they take in? Bright orange wedge shapes and glistening crisp edges? With your eyes on the fries, where's your mind? Is it on the fries too? I don't mean *thinking* about fries (*They aren't healthy but they taste SO good...*). I'm talking about a mutually attentive moment where your mental awareness is in sync with your eyes, so the seeing of fries is the focus of your mind as it's happening. Another way to explain this is, making a conscious choice to bring your mind to the sensory experience you're having with food as you're eating. It's mind and body aligned, and while it sounds obvious because the instructions are so simple, it's not usually how we consume food. Sometimes the mind syncs up with the senses as they interact with fries. But often it wanders off on tangents, like who's overdoing it with the ketchup.

Generally speaking, we overemphasize the thinking part of eating while underobserving and underdeveloping the experiential aspects of food. Popular blogs and social media feeds have a lot to say on this matter. They guide parents to say things like rainbow-colored veggies and fruits help the body in different ways or that cucumbers are "anytime foods" while cookies are "sometimes foods." Of course, there's nothing wrong with teaching kids age-appropriate nutrition basics. The problem is when that teaching focuses primarily on thinking about food, or exerting mental effort around how or what we eat. There's a big difference between doling out nutrition facts and helping your child mature as an eater.

Thinking about food (or yourself as an eater) is not the most important part of eating. Thinking about how and what you eat happens above your eyebrow line. We need more below-the-brow eating. Especially when talking to kids about food! This means being present for the sight, smell, touch, flavor, and sound arising with food. Five senses–based eating doesn't mean leaving your brain behind while you eat. It's about intentionally bringing your mind to what's happening in your body in the moment. Your five senses are the doorways to that, and it just so happens that kids are stellar at eating like this when given the opportunity.

Kids attune to five-senses exploration of eating with relative ease. That's because (as you recall from chapter 4) they start out eating mindfully and over time learn to bypass their innate curiosity, due at least in part to conditioning they receive around food. Awareness of the senses while eating is the natural entry point for helping kids eat better, because your five senses are the channels you use to experience food. When you intentionally pause, if only for a second, to unite your eyes and mind during a moment of eating, that sparks gastronomic intelligence.

You have the power to inspire this awareness in your child with new table talk. Mindfully coaching your child's observation of their five senses as they eat activates a kind of openness and possibility during meals. It doesn't guarantee your kid will eat things—especially things that don't bring them joy—but even a kid having a strong sensory feeling might not melt down when cued differently.

New Table Talk Cues

A simple building block for new table talk is to focus on one of the senses. Sight, smell, touch, sound, or flavor are great fodder for open-ended questions. Notice how I say "flavor," not "taste." The words "taste" and "flavor" are not synonymous in table talk terms: asking about flavor is preferable to asking your child about taste, because even if you mean "taste" as a nonthreatening noun ("the taste of food"), your child can hear it as a dreaded verb: as in "Taste it." Taste is an action. Flavor is an experience that includes smell, texture, temperature, and taste of food. So as we go along, you'll notice new table talk generally doesn't ask kids how things taste. That's intentional because the word "taste" inhibits how many kids explore food.

Paying attention to the five senses while eating is important because it's your child's lived experience with food. What they feel, hear, smell, see, and touch while eating are things that get neglected (or even vetoed) by old table talk ("It's just a little bit of sauce" or "But it's not even spicy!

If you try it a bunch, you get used to new flavors"). Tuning in to your senses is how you figure out what's working and what's not with food. It's also how you recognize when you want more of something or when you're full. All this happens for kids while they eat; we just don't ask them about it. Teaching your child five senses–based eating using new table talk empowers something essential for them: a sense of self-worth and agency with food. You are showing your child how to look inward and strengthen invaluable skills like self-trust and satisfaction as an eater.

Five senses–based eating makes more sense doing it than just reading about it. So try the next practice with your child. (This works best for kids age 3 and up). You'll need one small piece of fresh fruit per person. A single blueberry, a small apple slice, or a chunk of melon will do. If your child is under the age of four, then cut anything round (like a grape or cherry) in half. Some people prefer to use dried fruit, like a raisin, but whatever you have on hand will work. You might ask your child what fruit to use and explain to them that this practice is for both of you to notice whatever you can about what happens while you eat.

EXERCISE: Five-Senses Eating

Sit down with your child and one bite-size piece of fruit for each of you. If you're new to mindfulness or mindful eating, it can be helpful to do this exercise with the audio recording available at http://www.newharbinger. com/49463. Alternatively, you can read the directions below out loud, pacing yourself so your child can participate fully. If you read aloud, go step-by-step and wait (as best you can) to talk about things until after you finish the exercise. Be sure to take pauses between actions and between steps. Start reading out loud now:

Feel your body sitting in this chair…Notice your breathing…Air coming in and air going out—from your nose, chest, and belly.

Now focusing your eyes on the food…Using your fingers, pick it up…Take a close look…Seeing the color, the shape, and the texture of this food…What do you notice about this food with your eyes and fingers?

Bring the food up to your nose...Smelling it—what do you notice?... Take one more sniff...

Where is your mind at this moment?...Is it here with the smelling?...If not, gently bring your attention back to what's going on with your nose right now. Smelling, seeing, and touching this food are a few of the many ways you can experience it.

Looking at this food again...Wondering where it lived when it was growing...Imagine it warmed by the sun...washed by the rain...and resting under moonbeams at night.

This food took a trip to get to you...Imagining that journey in your mind...thankful for this food.

Now bring the food up to your lips and put it in your mouth... Closing your eyes if you'd like...Feel this one tiny piece of food, resting on your tongue...Don't chew it yet.

What's going on in your mouth right now?...Feeling the food and any changes.

If you're thinking about something else right now, just come back to the feeling in your mouth.

Chewing the food now...Feeling your jaw, tongue, and teeth... Listening to the sound of this food.

As you swallow, feel this food sliding down your throat...Noticing where this food is now.

Take a breath in and let it out...Now open your eyes if they're closed.

After you finish this practice of eating mindfully, spend a few minutes debriefing with your child. Ask about their experience and share what you noticed too. Take turns answering these questions:

- How was that for you?

- What did you notice?

- What happened in your eyes? How about your nose, mouth, ears, and mind?

- What was the most interesting thing about eating like this?

- What did you learn? What felt silly?

- How does paying attention like this help you when you eat?

The purpose of this exercise isn't to start eating meals in slow motion cued by tedious steps. It's to activate awareness of your mind and whole-body senses with food. Kids are innately good at this. It's old table talk that stifles their process. That means your job as parent is to notice what's happening while you eat and give voice to that with new table talk.

Five senses–based eating doesn't require extra resources. Your senses are already present and active while you eat. The new part is consciously bringing your attention to what's going on between your senses and food while you eat and, when your awareness takes commercial breaks, returning to your senses over and over again.

What to Do About a Wandering Mind

During the mindful eating, did your mind wander? Even several times? That's normal. It doesn't mean you're bad at mindful eating or that five senses–based eating doesn't work for you and your child. It means you're human, with a mind that thinks. Remember, thinking isn't bad; it's just not the skill we're trying to strengthen around food. Your awareness might show up and peel off again eighty-five times during one measly snack. That's okay. You're not doing it wrong. In fact, you're right on track. This mindfulness practice is about *what you do when you notice your mind is distracted*, that split-second moment when you realize your mind is on email or laundry instead of the flaky, tender croissant dissolving on your tongue.

When you recognize you're lost in thought, simply pause. You've successfully realized you were away. That's the whole point! As Zen master Thich Nhat Hahn teaches, you've now got a choice about how to proceed. You can simply begin again by bringing your attention back to the food or sensations right here in your nose, eyes, ears, or mouth. Intentionally notice one sense or another, and bring your mind to that. This is why mindful eating is called a "practice." It's not a tactic or a strategy. It's all about coming back, once you notice your mind has wandered. Time and again, practice returning to the present moment as you're eating.

But why do all this? If you're up to your eyeballs in food struggles, can five senses–based eating really help? The answer is yes, it's worth trying because it reduces the odds of a meltdown. When you tune in to your senses while you eat—and work from that angle as a parent—you tend your child's process of eating instead of examining their plate. Each time you start judging how or what they're eating, you come back to noticing your senses because, in that instant, you find better ground to operate from. This is a big shift from how most people handle food woes with kids. Best of all, it's free, you can do it anywhere, and it takes less time than you think. Let's take a closer look at how five senses–based eating helps kids (and parents!) with food struggles.

How Kids Eat

Six-year-old Sadie is good at noticing things, like how she hates brussels sprouts. Spotting a dish of these at dinner, she frowns and says, "Brussels sprouts are really gross." Her mom replies with new table talk: "Which part? Tell me what you see with brussels sprouts."

Go back and reread Sadie's complaint, and read her mom's response out loud. Can you hear how new table talk doesn't shy away from the problem? In fact, it probes a little deeper, inviting the reality of the situation to be expressed. There's good reason for doing this, on both macro and micro levels: it strengthens Sadie's gastronomic intelligence (a big deal) by pulling up a seat for the food struggle (small potatoes). I got an email from Sadie's mom after they started five senses–based eating. She wanted to update me on what Sadie was saying about brussels sprouts: "They have a low taste. Strong and dark on my tongue. Not like pineapple. That's a high and bright flavor, with juice. Brussels sprouts aren't like that."

Sadie's sharing a lot from her senses about brussels sprouts. She doesn't love them in her mouth, but her mind and the rest of her senses are wide open to exploring. Her mom helped that happen by using new table talk phrases. But how does encouraging Sadie's use of her five senses prevent her from freaking out over food? To understand that, we need to explore further how kids eat.

Kids experiences of food aren't as fixed as you might think. And even when their habits seem unchangeable, it doesn't help kids when you point that out to them. We tend to think about how kids eat in terms of foods they like or foods they dislike, which is an oversimplification. There are even rating scales and food apps for kids extolling this approach. One Tinder-style app shows pictures of vegetables that kids swipe left or right to record how they feel about that food. This reduces something rich and complex (like multisensory observations of food) to one reactive and reductive opinion. It's a snapshot in time, when the real food with its touch, sight, smell, sound, and flavor potential isn't even available to be considered. This doesn't help kids with food. It only tells you what they think about pictures of food at any given moment in time, which is nothing like kids observing or experiencing food using their senses.

It's risky to teach kids that food and eating are one-dimensional like that, because it's win or lose with nothing in between. Talk about a scenario ripe for meltdowns! Imagine what would have happened if Sadie's mom had replied, "You haven't had this kind of brussels sprouts before" or "You have to take two bites before you can say you don't like them" or "Eat them anyway!" Instead, her open-ended question about brussels sprouts acknowledged her kid's experience and made that a stepping-stone for dealing with this food rejection. Your options for engaging kids with food are jeopardized when you or your kids believe food and how you experience it are static decisions. Food is dynamic, diverse, and sensorial. Even stuff you don't like! Approaches to food that disregard the five senses fail to engage kids as eaters. And even worse, they cut off kids' natural inclination to be curious and connected while eating.

Kids have much more to say about food then "yuck" or "yum." They know gooey and juicy. Kids know creamy. They know salty, sticky, and chewy. *Our table talk needs to help kids access and believe in their inner wisdom and experiences around food.* Kids relish the chance to engage in mindful eating, especially when given the gift of time and space to share their observations. This is what the Table Talk Method is about. It's an introspective process you champion with your child while they eat. When you feed the heart and soul of your child as an eater, you help them access something bigger and more significant: gastronomic intelligence.

Gastronomic Intelligence

Gastronomic intelligence is the inward compass you consult (consciously or unconsciously) to find your way with food, whether you're a kid or an adult. It's your inner wisdom and awareness of eating. It's the internal witness and resource that senses who you are and what you need from food. It's not how smart or savvy you are about nutrition choices but your felt sense of food and eating observations as they arise. It's knowing how and what to eat to satisfy your needs, and it's clear seeing of the mental chatter that bubbles up to judge those behaviors.

Gastronomic intelligence is an intrinsic attribute that everyone has the capacity to strengthen. It's particularly accessible for kids because they haven't learned to *should* on themselves with food. GI is important because it steers the ship of eating over a lifetime. And table talk (old or new) is the most direct way parents affect GI in kids. Gastronomic intelligence evolves as kids integrate what they're told about themselves as eaters (your table talk) with their direct and personal experiences of eating as felt through their five senses.

Gastronomic intelligence has three components related to food: satisfaction, self-trust, and self-compassion. *Satisfaction* is choosing and eating food that gives you comfort or pleasure. *Self-trust* is believing in your ability to make those choices and allowing yourself to fully experience enjoyment from food without fear, judgment, or overthinking things. *Self-compassion* is knowing how to be kind to yourself about eating. This means when the little voice inside your head chastises you for how or what you're eating, you don't get hung up, unequivocally believing that one-sided message. You learn to respond to unhelpful self-talk about eating with the same kindness you would offer a dear friend.

Gastronomic intelligence might sound like a tall order for a little kid. Not to mention for you as a parent, trying to help it evolve! Besides, isn't this book about ending mealtime meltdowns? The main thing to know is that gastronomic intelligence is the sense of self-worth and assuredness with food that is everyone's birthright as an eater. It's your deepest sense of being okay, just as you are, while you eat. If you don't currently feel so okay or worthy as an eater, I want to help.

My mission as a mindfulness-based dietitian/nutritionist is helping people connect with and nurture their gastronomic intelligence, because gastronomic intelligence is present even when it feels hidden. Everyone has this type of intelligence, even people who might be referred to (or consider themselves) "picky." Gastronomic intelligence has nothing to do with excellence around food. It's how well you connect with your internal witness to process eating experiences for yourself. That's why it's such an integral part of resolving food conflict.

GI and Food Struggles

At first, GI might seem flowery and abstract. How on earth can this concept help you stop food fights with your kid? Gastronomic intelligence is the bull's-eye on the proverbial target you need to aim for when feeding kids, because GI is the resource your child uses to work through their observations of food. When table talk ignores or opposes GI, it aggravates kids while they eat. It causes them to feel discord that can materialize into a tailspin. The more kids freak out about food, the more parents use old table talk or, frankly, give up—either of which make things worse. Old table talk and throwing in the towel yield the same result. They both lead kids further away from their gastronomically intelligent core. Navigating a mealtime meltdown without the aid of gastronomic intelligence is like trying to row a boat after your paddle fell in the water. You're stuck, it's stressful, and you can't generate any momentum.

New table talk guides your child to eat by tuning in to gastronomic intelligence. When your words are informed by GI, you stop misfiring during meals. New table talk anchors your child to the awareness they need to work through food-related distress. It's the smoothest and fastest way out of mealtime drama. So how do you nurture gastronomic intelligence?

Gastronomic intelligence doesn't come from reading a book, even this book! It comes from within. That's why your parenting around food is so critical. Kids naturally eat with their five senses, but they need your words to stay tuned, digest, and integrate their observations to make meaning. Your job is to relate to your child as they eat using communication skills that guide them to tap into their gastronomic intelligence. Kids' GI is already intact. You're not creating it. New table talk is the pointer that helps your child access and eat from this place of awareness.

In *The Eating Instinct*, Virginia Sole-Smith says, "Eating well cannot be about following the rules; it has to be about trusting our own instincts, which value safety, comfort, and pleasure just as much as nutrition, and sometimes more" (2018, xiv). This quote speaks to the magnitude and importance of gastronomic intelligence and the need for us as parents to help kids learn to trust those instincts with food.

How to Foster GI

Right now, you come to the table hoping your kid will eat a little something "healthy," (however you define that). Your child comes to mealtime hungry for a little sense of sovereignty (however they experience that). This dynamic fanned with old typical table talk doesn't allow for true cooperation. It causes both you and your child to double down to get what you want with food. When you change the focus to what your kid is sensing or noticing as they eat, you land on the mutually beneficial playing field of gastronomic intelligence. This is where everyone can get in the game.

There are three main ways to foster gastronomic intelligence in kids:

1. Practice five senses–based eating with your child.

2. Describe food using adjectives, not dichotomous labels like "good" and "bad."

3. Ask more than you tell kids about their eating.

You've already learned how to engage the five senses while eating with your child, which is a cornerstone of the Table Talk Method. Now we'll add some new communication skills. First, we'll discuss how to expand your gastronomic vocabulary with the power of adjectives. Then you'll learn how to use what parents rank as their number one new table talk phrase—it's four short words that iron out lots of food troubles. The third method for nurturing gastronomic intelligence (ask more than you tell while you eat) is covered in chapter 6.

Expand Your Gastronomic Vocabulary

Eating from a five-senses perspective gives you and your child new insights about food, and it's important to talk about that! In this section you'll learn how to talk with your child about food using expressive adjectives, or descriptive words. This can be anything you notice about food while you eat, like its color, texture, temperature, smell, sound, sight, or flavor. The purpose is to teach your child to describe their experiences of food, which leads to new outcomes. Here's a quick list of adjectives kids have come up with when parents used new table talk in tandem with five senses–based eating.

Sight: fluffy, wet, lumpy, steamy, greasy, jiggly

Smell: minty, fishy, fresh, vinegary, garlicky, lemony

Flavor: juicy, spicy, tangy, sweet, salty, sour

Touch: crusty, silky, stringy, mushy, gooey, dry

Sound: crunchy, fizzy, slurpy, chewy, gritty, sticky

The reason to get kids talking about food using adjectives is simple: it gives you something practical to work with when things unravel during meals. Using adjectives to describe what your five senses get from food also strengthens gastronomic intelligence, so you're simultaneously diffusing volatility while you help your child develop skills of healthy eating.

It's important to choose adjectives that capture your *sensory experiences of food* and not adjectives that infer morality or value judgments (like "good" and "bad") with food. For example, "disgusting" and "delicious" are adjectives you might use to describe oatmeal, but they don't depict what your five senses took in (below your brow line) with that food. They tell me, categorically, what you *think* about oatmeal, but remember, thinking isn't what we're after. You're not teaching kids to size up their food. You're showing them how to turn inward and feel it. So if your kid says their food is "gross" or "disgusting" or even "delicious" or "yummy," encourage them with open-ended questions like "Which part?" "How so," or "Where's that feeling in your body?"

Kids can come up with worthwhile adjectives even when they don't eat a certain food. Think of Sadie and the brussels sprouts. Her mom's new table talk cued Sadie to consult her five senses while she interfaced with food. Then her mom could focus on listening, which leads to far less conflict than old table talk.

It's true that talking about food using adjectives is a subjective matter. But that's the point. No one is "picky" or melting down over food in a vacuum. It's idiosyncratic stuff! To work through difficulties, your kid needs some agency and you need something tangible to work with besides "I love it" or "I hate it" with food. So, here's to adjectives! They're quintessentially curious, and the best part of using them in your table talk is hearing what your kids come up with in return. I love the words kids concoct when talking about their sensory experiences of food. Ezra, age six, is a fan of lasagna due to its "zingy" flavor! And Nabil, the eight-year-old son of a client, describes his cereal as "crisp-ish."

EXERCISE: Use Adjectives in Table Talk

The new table talk prompts below help you ramp up on adjectives. When using them with your child, choose one of the five senses at a time. Fill in the blank with whatever makes most sense in the moment. Falafel is the example here, but you can adapt these prompts for any food:

1. How's the falafel _____? (Fill in the blank with *smell, look, feel,* or *sound.*)

2. What kind of _____ [*flavors, smells, sounds,* or *textures*] does falafel have?

3. Tell me about the _____ [*look, smell, feel, sound,* or *flavor*] of falafel for you.

With very young kids who are still learning names of food, you can offer, as an example, "This is falafel. For me, it's warm and crispy." Follow that by asking your child, "How's the falafel feel for you?" Or shortened, "How does it feel?" Even if your child is still learning to speak, don't skip asking what they observe. They don't need to respond in words, and they don't need to answer at all. Sharing and soliciting adjectives is important, regardless of a child's verbal skills.

Modify the sophistication of your new table talk to match your child's maturity, but keep the emphasis on *the act of noticing* what they see, smell, touch, hear, and taste with food. It's not necessary for kids to actually eat something to benefit from or identify adjectives. "What do you notice about falafel?" could be color, texture, or temperature, as noticed through the eyes or felt with fingers. This fosters gastronomic intelligence.

A second way to incorporate adjectives into your table talk is when your child asks for a specific food. This is your opportunity to use an adjective-enhanced reply. If your child wants yogurt, for example, you could say, "You want cold, smooth, and sweet." As the parent, you get to decide if it's time to eat and if yogurt is an option. If so, serve the yogurt along with the adjective-inclusive table talk. If it's not snack time or yogurt isn't an option, you still need those adjectives. They create better table talk! If yogurt isn't on the menu, you can say, "Yogurt isn't available right now. Cold, smooth, or sweet options are a pear or grapes." This new table talk grounds kids in gastronomic intelligence and teaches greater flexibility with food. It might also help you avoid fighting over yogurt.

Yogurt isn't the only workable thing if what your child wants is something cold, smooth or sweet—and you're not using adjectives to dupe your child or pull a bait and switch. You're maintaining charge of what food is served while inviting your child to choose a snack using their internal compass. This is how adjectives help kids cooperate around food—not cooperate as in comply but as in *collaborate*—so your job as feeder and theirs as eater both have room at the table. New table talk establishes new precedents. Instead of a battle of wills, you and your child work together using adjectives.

Paying Attention to Internal Cues

Teaching your child to use adjectives with food also helps them listen to their body while they eat. *Listen to your body while you eat* may be amorphous advice, but I'm saying it to point out there are specific ways you can teach your child to pay attention to internal cues. Using adjectives and practicing five senses–based eating show kids how to satisfy themselves with food. The more they do this as children, the easier it will be for them as adults to find food they want, enjoy what they eat, and know how much will do the trick. These are skills your child develops when your table talk is oriented toward gastronomic intelligence. GI is the part of you that's talking when you listen to your body while you eat.

Adjectives enrich how your child relates to food, even when that feels pestilent. My friend Amy took her five-year-old hiking. She packed granola for a snack. When her daughter lost steam, Amy broke out the bag and tossed a nutty, crunchy, cluster into her mouth (see what I did with adjectives just then?). Her daughter, quite hangry, asserted defiantly, "Granola IS NOT a good snack!" Cue the wilderness meltdown (preferable to the airplane or restaurant version but aggravating nonetheless). Granola is all they had. Before you judge Amy as a rookie who should've just packed five different snacks, let's be honest: if you really want to end food battles, the way out can't be a backpack full of food. Stuck in the woods with a kvetching kid made Amy a little ornery herself, so she said, "Wow! This granola is so soft and chewy."

"THIS?!" exclaimed her daughter, grabbing a hunk and hoisting it overhead.

"Yes," Amy continued, "kind of like a gummy bear." Her daughter popped the granola in her mouth, then amplified her crunching to prove the point. How clever! Rather than plead with her daughter to eat, Amy used adjectives, which prompted her daughter to explore for herself—using gastronomic intelligence.

Obviously, being goofy or contrary like this depends on your child's mood and age. But adjectives even help grown-ups try new foods, and you can adjust new table talk for maturity. With older kids ask, "What's the difference between bitter, pungent, and astringent foods?" Or based on your child's age, watch *Waffles + Mochi* or *Salt Fat Acid Heat*. These shows are a window into a world of flavor without even leaving your couch! You can also try a game I call, "Guess Three Ingredients," which is just like it sounds. Kids try to name three ingredients in whatever they're eating using the tools inherently at work, their full array of senses relating to food.

Along these same lines is Jan Chozen Bays's concept of the *nine types of hunger*. Bays is a pediatrician, Zen master, mindful-eating instructor, and the author of *Mindful Eating*. She teaches the difference between eye hunger, touch hunger, nose hunger, ear hunger, mouth hunger, stomach hunger, cellular hunger, heart hunger, and mind hunger. Did you know there were so many kinds of hunger? I recommend exploring these types of hunger with your child and for yourself, because they are direct pathways for nurturing gastronomic intelligence.

You can try this enlightening practice now, as Bays has graciously allowed me to adapt the "Basic Mindful Eating Meditation" from her book (2017). Grab a raisin or another small piece of food for each member of your family, and then try this eating meditation together.

Basic Mindful Eating Meditation

This exercise guides your understanding of the nine types of hunger, bringing gastronomic intelligence to life in new ways.

1. Begin by sitting quietly and assessing your baseline hunger. How hungry are you on a scale of 0 to 10? Where do you "look" in your body to decide how hungry you are?

2. Imagine that you are a scientist on a mission to explore a new planet. As you walk around, you find a small object and pick it up. Place the raisin (or other food item) on your palm. You are going to investigate it with the tools you have, your five senses. You have no idea what this object is. You have never seen it before.

3. Eye hunger: First you investigate this object with your eyes. Look at its color, shape, and surface texture. What does the mind say it could be? Now rate your eye hunger for this item. On a scale of 0 to 10, how much hunger do you have for this object based on what your eyes see?

4. Nose hunger: Now you investigate it with your nose. Smell it, refresh the nose, and sniff it again. Does this change your idea of whether it might be edible? Now rate your nose hunger. On a scale of 0 to 10, how much hunger do you have for this object based on what your nose smells?

5. Mouth hunger: Now you investigate this object with your mouth. Place it in your mouth, but do not bite it. You can roll it around and explore it with the tongue. What do you notice?

Now you can bite this mysterious object, but only once. After biting it once, roll it around again in the mouth, and explore it with the tongue. What do you notice?

Now rate mouth hunger. On a scale of 0 to 10, how much hunger do you have for this object based upon what the mouth tastes and feels? In other words, how much does the mouth want to experience more of it?

6. Stomach hunger: Now you decide to take a risk and eat this unknown object. You chew it slowly, noticing the changes in the mouth in texture and taste. You swallow it. You notice whether there are still any bits in the mouth. What does the tongue do when you have finished eating it? How long can you detect the flavor?

   Now rate stomach hunger. Is the stomach full or not, satisfied or not? On a scale of 0 to 10, rate stomach hunger. In other words, how much does the stomach want more of this food?

7. Cellular hunger: Become aware of this food passing into the body. Absorption begins as soon as we begin chewing. Are there any sensations that tell you that this food is being absorbed? How is it being received by the cells in the body? Now rate cellular hunger. On a scale of 0 to 10, how much would the cells like to have more of this food?

8. Mind hunger: Can you hear what the mind is saying about this food? (Hint: Often the mind talks in *shoulds* or *should nots*.) Now rate mind hunger. On a scale of 0 to 10, how much would the mind like you to have more of this food?

9. Heart hunger: Is the heart saying anything about this food? On a scale of 0 to 10, how soothing or comforting is this food? Would the heart like you to have more of this food?

The unique thing about this eating meditation is how it helps you feel the ways and places hunger shows up. Spoiler alert—it's not just your belly! This is eye-opening for many adults, but kids often feel it straightaway.

Maybe not every hunger type clicks with you, but the activation of gastro-nomic intelligence is real. GI is where you go to get information about how hungry and full you are (and most other details about eating). I meet many adult clients suffering from the same deficiency: not knowing or believing they have GI in the first place. They mistakenly conclude they lack will power around food and aren't good-enough eaters, due to "out-of-control" portions or their inability to "stay away from certain foods." That's toxic diet culture talking (a topic too broad to cover here). But the antidote to all that banter is strengthening gastronomic intelligence. The nine types of hunger work wonders for that.

Use adjectives to describe food and your senses while eating, and ask your child questions so they do the same. Make your words as simple or elaborate as your child needs. When they ask for a certain food, weave an adjective into your reply and explore as many of the nine types of hunger as you can when eating with your child. (New table talk on this topic is coming up in chapter 8). You're consciously nurturing your child's inner compass of eating with these simple steps. Many parents I work with are astonished to learn even reluctant eaters have a lot to say about foods once adjective-rich new table talk is introduced.

Kids Speaking Their Minds

What descriptive words does your child come up with when asked a gastronomically intelligent question about the sight, smell, sound, or feel of food? Emma, age nine, says "Pink Lady apples are my favorite because they're hard, crunchy, and sweet. When I take a bite, it holds up in my mouth. Apples that dissolve in that mushy way don't do it for me." Gastronomic intelligence is deeply experiential like that. It's more spe-cific than surface-level like or dislike. The descriptive words Emma uses recount her sensory experience. She's acquainted with apples in a way that goes beyond just favorites. Emma using adjectives (crunchy, hard, and sweet) shows her inner awareness. She's mindfully using her five senses with apples, both the ones she prefers and the ones she dislikes.

This is gastronomic intelligence in action. Emma's bringing this kind of awareness to eating is a skill she needs for the rest of her life. And she's got the hang of it at nine years old! She's eating guided by her internal compass, which, her parents report, "has been the only thing to make a dent in her finicky eating."

The change in how Emma engages with food happened because her parents adopted new table talk. They mindfully choose what they say to Emma about her eating while she's at it. They consciously use questions, not critiques. They don't highlight things they wish she'd change. Their words help Emma practice part of her eating process out loud. This shifts family dynamics during meals. Displeasure with food doesn't trigger automatic reactions on the part of Emma or her parents. Some meals are easier than others, but even when food frustration arises, Emma's parents are confident in their new table talk. Their words energize Emma's gastronomic intelligence, which leads to fewer face-offs over food.

Imagine Emma, ten or twenty years from now, choosing what to eat self-assuredly. Having practiced GI skills since she was a kid, she'll know how to figure out which food and how much it awakens inner pleasure. Satisfaction, self-trust, and self-compassion (the three pillars of gastronomic intelligence) are baked right in to how Emma's learning to eat every day. But you might be thinking, *My kid's not like Emma...*

When Kids Eat "Mostly Junk"

My client Donna was leery of five senses–based eating because she worried it might heighten her child's cravings for packaged foods. Logan, age eleven, wants salty, crunchy snacks "all day long," and Donna worries these foods have an addictive quality that might get stronger if she encourages curiosity.

I understand Donna's fear that eating with greater awareness could lead to more cravings, but the research on mindful eating suggests just the opposite. Mindful eating reduces overeating and improves people's relationship with food (Zervos et al. 2021). It also reduces impulsive food choice in adolescents (Hendrickson and Rasmussen 2017). Becoming aware of your eating from moment to moment (not judging by thinking but noticing with your senses) allows greater discernment of pleasure as well as increased wisdom to know if a food is or isn't doing it for you. Don Gerrard, author of *One Bowl*, calls this "food that hums" (2001, 100). When food is aligned with your inner needs and desires, it gives you the same feeling as humming. A light, soothing, vibrational delight you get from savoring food. That's how five senses–based eating works for, not against, your child. It's another skill you teach them to practice: how to notice experiences with food—even "junk food"—bite by bite to decide if, how, and when it's providing satisfaction (humming) or not. Sometimes the alternative is eating the whole bag or stopping only when guilt and discomfort arise.

Gastronomic intelligence is a reliable, inner compass everyone has as an eater. Your job as a parent is to help your child access and get to know that place while they eat, whether they love or hate the food. It works either way. Food woes can come out of nowhere for a million different reasons, but what you can do about it isn't as elusive as it seems. Bring your five senses and adjectives to dinner. These are tools you can use to help your kids deal with food troubles. When kids say food is "good," "bad," or "gross," you can ask, "Like what?" "Like how?" or "Which part?" Try to get your child describing what their five senses pick up on with food. Model this by sharing one or two adjectives based on your own experience. Use short and simple new table talk like "For me, this is salty and tart." Then ask, "How's the flavor for you?"

Five senses–based eating and talking in adjectives diffuse meltdown risk, which brings us to that all-star new phrase I mentioned earlier. It's four simple words: "What would help it?"

The Add-On Method

"What would help it?" is new table talk that kicks off a method I call *the add-on*. The add-on is a two-step approach to deal with food resistance and rejection in kids. I first published this in October 2019 on a website called Fatherly.com.

The add-on consists of the new table talk phrase "What would help it?" along with a supply of condiment-like foods kids can sprinkle, squeeze, dip, or add to what's on their plate. Add-on foods include fresh or dried herbs and spices, crushed nuts or cereals, and an assortment of dips and dressings. Things like cinnamon, unsweetened shredded coconut, fresh lemon or lime wedges. Other options might be mustard, hummus, or a dollop of sour cream. Add-ons are condiments, not meal replacements.

To implement the add-on, keep two or three small containers of add-on foods in the fridge or a cabinet, somewhere your child can reach with your permission. Some parents label these containers with a sticker or masking tape that says "add-on," then line them up in the door of the fridge for easy access. Enlist your child in choosing and preparing a few add-ons to keep at the ready.

Now you're prepared for your child to reject food. When they freak out about tofu, you ask, "What would help it?" When they say, "Nothing!" You stick with your new table talk questions like "What's the texture of tofu?" or "What happens when you poke tofu with a chopstick?" Listen to what your child says without trying to convince them of anything. Then (if needed) repeat your new phrase again, "What would help it?" These words cue your child to get an add-on if they choose.

When you first introduce this method, you need to explain to your child how it works. Don't make a big speech, but just say something like this to your child the next time food resistance arises:

"What's one thing that might help this food?" Wait to hear what your kid says. Then say, "That's called an *add-on*. It's like a topping you can choose to help food work better for you. Add-ons we have right now are: crushed cereal, mustard, or coconut flakes." List a few options you have on hand.

Use the add-on method as often as needed, because it's impossible to meet your child's precise food wishes and demands constantly. I bet you too have made their favorite sandwich, then somehow cut it wrong?! You'd be amazed what new table talk ("What would help it?") can do for those jagged little edges.

If your child rejects add-ons, stick with other new table talk like, "What do you notice?" or "Tell me about…" You can also say, "You don't have to eat it," but whatever comes after that must uphold and not jeopardize that promise. This means sometimes repeating the same new table talk phrases. It's okay to use words that feel redundant. Consider them as new table talk guardrails helping you not drift away from your child's direct experience.

You can't control a kid who's freaking out about food, but you can use new table talk to point them in the direction of what they need to eke out a solution. Your newest phrase, "What would help it?" leads kids inward to decide what (if anything) from the available options jives with their gastronomic intelligence. Take refuge in your five senses, sharing an adjective or two. From there, use new table talk that directs your child to do the same. This is how you reduce meltdowns, moment by moment, with responsive words that help kids cope when they're feeling overwhelmed about food. Forcing your child to try a food is never advisable, but you can ask them a question to enliven curiosity or connection. And then you can listen. Ask. Then listen, actively. That's the new table talk way.

How you eat with your child and how you talk to them about their eating are currently undergoing major renovations. The new vocabulary you're building enables your child to draw upon their gastronomic intelligence. This is better and vastly different from hoping they just swallow some broccoli. You're training your child with skills of healthy eating, so they can figure out *what would help* when they aren't psyched about dinner.

Let's test your learning from this chapter by returning to an exercise you did in chapter 2 where you explored your table talk. In that exercise, you imagined having dinner with your child and how you would respond to them making different statements about the food in front of them. It's time for you to do this exercise again, but this time bolstered by your new table talk knowledge and phrases.

EXERCISE: Practice New Table Talk

This exercise involves talking out loud and takes a few minutes. At the top of a clean page in your journal, write "My New Table Talk." Then read one of the following statements at a time, pretending your child is saying this to you, and respond aloud with new table talk, such as "What would help it?" "What do you notice?" "Tell me about…" As an example, imagine your child says, "I don't like asparagus!" You could say, "What would help it?" or create a question based on the five senses like, "How does the asparagus _____?" (Fill in the blank with smell, look, feel, or sound). Take a few rounds responding aloud to each of the following statements to get a good feel for new table talk.

What do you say when your child says this?

1. "I don't like asparagus."

2. "I don't want green beans."

3. "I *hate* tofu."

4. "I don't like apples anymore."

5. "Why do we ALWAYS have to eat salad?"

6. "But I *did* try it, and I still don't like it!"

What new table talk did you use? Write it in your journal, especially new phrases that have an "Aha!" quality for you. This is the beginning of your customized new table talk, and there's much more to come.

Once you've written down some new table talk, turn back in your journal to find your original answers to the prompts in chapter 2. Can you see and hear the difference between your old and new table talk?

Five senses–based eating and using adjectives in table talk are two of the main ways to strengthen gastronomic intelligence in your child. And nurturing GI is the most important goal when feeding kids. Using new table talk helps your child take their seat as an eater to experience satisfaction, trust, and compassion for themselves. That's how we all want to feel with food. And it's a teachable thing, even when a meltdown is looming. Curiosity and connection are the launchpad for your new table talk, and gastronomic intelligence is where you want it to land.

So ground your table talk in curiosity and connection. Sit down to eat with your five senses, and link your mind to your body's experience. From here, verbalize an adjective that captures your felt sense of a food, and follow that by asking your child to share what they notice too. Don't do this ad nauseam—the goal isn't constant chatter about food, rather it is about replacing what you used to say with fewer and more effective words. When things get dicey, stick with straightforward table talk like "What would help it?" keeping your child's gastronomic intelligence in mind as you talk to them while they eat. When that feels challenging (and I promise it will), remember the image of your young child that you consulted in the meet-your-eater quiz from chapter 4. That picture of this kid, eating when they were a baby, eating with everything they've got. You're doing all you can, too, to connect with them and make food and eating better for both of you. With that in mind, let's turn to the nitty-gritty of what to say.

CHAPTER 6

Build a Foundation for What to Say

Eight-year-old Olivia is a messy eater. Her fingers function as her utensil of choice, and she wears spaghetti sauce on her cheeks and chin until the single swipe of a napkin signals the end of her meal. Alongside the food she's eating, Oliva regularly absorbs an earful of old table talk, aimed at whipping up some semblance of manners. "Olivia," her mother pleads. "You're eating like a pig! Please use your fork." Unfazed by etiquette, Oliva fully embodies her eating experiences.

"You need to *stop* eating with your hands," chides her father. "It's just disgusting!"

Exasperated and embarrassed, Olivia's well-intentioned parents are baffled about how to influence her eating behavior. Their efforts to improve her technique have done little to shift her habits, and their style of coaching has developed an urgent edge.

"It's one thing for a toddler to eat this way," laments Olivia's mother, "but she's in third grade!"

I met Olivia's family through her grandmother Joyce, who works as a lunch monitor at an elementary school nearby. Joyce assists kids opening milk cartons, handing out condiments, and providing a general sort of comfort and order in the cafeteria. Struck by students' widespread tendency to stuff, scarf, and gulp their food, Joyce sought my advice about how to help young eaters, most notably Olivia, to "improve her manners."

I quizzed Joyce with what has become my archetypal question: "What do you say to Olivia while she's eating?" Chewing on my query, Joyce eventually replied: "Olivia, why don't you try using your fork?

Eating with your hands isn't very polite. If you don't use a fork, people will think you're rude."

Joyce's phrases might sound familiar from the types of table talk we discussed in chapter 3. Her attempts to help Olivia include a closed-ended question followed by corrective and conditional table talk. These phrases pose problems when coaching how kids eat. They're meant to convey valuable lessons and offer helpful cues, but in typical fashion, they backfire because kids ignore commands to fix how they eat and perhaps misconstrue what's been said, so what they hear instead is: "You're bad," "You're wrong," or "You're awful at eating." It's hard to motivate anyone to change if your pointers insinuate inadequacy.

I suggested Joyce try an entirely different approach, asking Olivia to describe what it feels like as she eats with her hands, to ask, "What's the feeling of spaghetti on your fingers?" or "How do those noodles feel?" I reminded Joyce to ask these questions from a place of sincere curiosity, avoiding any hint of disapproval or condescension in her tone. The aim was for Joyce to ask open-ended questions to elicit descriptive words from Olivia about her sensory experience, as she feels the spaghetti with her hands. Joyce was genuinely puzzled by this advice. She nodded her head slowly, trying these words on in her mind. Then her eyes met mine, and she muttered, "*Okay...*but what should I expect Olivia to say?" I have no idea of what Olivia might say, and that's the point! Contrary to how we usually feed kids, the Table Talk Method involves asking kids, not telling them, about their eating experiences.

In this chapter, you'll learn about five different communication styles. These include four types of questions—open-ended, closed-ended, prove-it, and probing questions—and reflective statements. I'll teach you which of these makes effective new table talk and which to avoid, because intentionally using or limiting these words is the center-piece of building your new table talk.

This chapter is chock-full of new table talk and explanations for why these words work. You'll become a question aficionado, pairing open-ended inquiries with reflective statements, so curiosity reclaims its right-ful seat at your table. Doing this prioritizes satisfaction and self-trust with food, which leads to less conflict around food and happier, healthier eaters.

We're all evolving as eaters, Olivia included. It's unlikely she'll eat with her hands forever, but while she's at it, her grandma and parents have a plan. They know what to say to guide Olivia's sensory exploration of food and help her tap into gastronomic intelligence. Her behavior still pushes their buttons, but new table talk helps them to ease up on Olivia and themselves during meals. Less reactivity is one way the Table Talk Method works. It does not eliminate dissonance but gives you better tools to manage the chaos. Tools like open-ended questions and reflective statements that don't put kids down as eaters. Asking "How's that different with a fork?" is the kind of simple tweak that got Olivia using utensils, without being told.

. I want to be clear. This isn't the same as kids playing with food. The Table Talk Method is your intentional use of specific communication skills to nurture curiosity and connectivity with your child as they eat. It's a kind of syncing up between you and your kid while eating and, more importantly, between kids, their food, and their innermost self as eaters. The skills you'll gain in this chapter energize a new kind of family meal, where well-defined questions guide kids' explorations of eating so they exercise gastronomic intelligence.

The shift I'm describing begins with understanding four basic types of questions. First let's dig into the difference between open- and closed-ended questions.

Open-Ended Questions

Open-ended questions get kids talking about their observations, feelings, and eating experiences in great detail. Phrased properly, these questions avoid leading or invoking judgment and aim to capture as much information about your child's eating as they're willing and able to share. Two open-ended prompts you've already learned are "What do you notice?" and "Tell me about…"

Open-ended questions spawn table talk wins. Questions like "What do you notice about red peppers?" or "How's the pear smell?" direct kids to their five senses, so they tune in to what's unfolding. Open-ended questions fuel intrigue and help kids take note of what's happening while they eat. They also guide kids to process those observations and deepen their innermost awareness with food.

Open-ended questions, also called "wondering questions," might sound like a no-brainer, but they're rare in typical table talk, and that's a big problem. We don't usually ask kids about their food and eating experiences while they eat. And when we do, the questions we ask are usually the least helpful, closed-ended kind, like "Did you try it yet?" or "Are you done eating?" When you steer clear of any category of old table talk and replace it with an open-ended question, you're transforming things for the better.

Asking your child "What do you notice about broccoli?" is an open-ended question. It puts the emphasis on intrigue, not probability of ingestion. A kid's answer to "What do you notice about broccoli?" can be anything, from "It's yucky!" to "Green and crunchy" to "Roasty and soft." The key is to string together a chain of open-ended questions, so your table talk helps your child dig in to what's going on for them with broccoli, right then and there. When your child says broccoli is "yucky," try another open-ended question, like "Which part?" Open-ended questions are like playing tennis. You want to keep returning the ball. Lob a light series of open-ended questions into your child's court. It's fundamental for raising healthy eaters. Open-ended questions become more obvious when you understand the closed-ended kind.

Closed-Ended Questions

Closed-ended questions evoke short, often one-word replies. They are typical of old table talk (see chapter 3). They cut off conversation and stifle your ability to actively listen to what your kids have to say about eating. Closed-ended questions such as "Do you like broccoli?" or "Have you tried the broccoli?" result in truncated answers like "No" and "I don't want to." Closed-ended questions shut down kids' curiosity with food, short-circuiting their stream of gastronomic intelligence. Even if your child isn't keen on eating broccoli (yet), they probably have observations and sensory experiences to tell you about broccoli if you ask the right kind of question.

"Have you tried the broccoli?" sounds innocuous and inviting, but it's useless for getting kids to engage with broccoli, because it's a closed-ended question. There are two probable answers to "Have you tried the broccoli?" Yes or no. Neither one promotes kids' exploring color, smell, texture, sound, or anything else about broccoli. Closed-ended questions coax terse replies and squash kids' curiosity as eaters. Closed-ended questions result in missed opportunities to activate curiosity and connection, and they fail to nurture kids' gastronomic intelligence.

How to Root Out Closed-Ended Questions

Avoid starting questions with these six words: "do," "did," "can," "will," "have," and "are." These verbs are usually glued to the word "you," as in: "Do you?" "Did you?" "Can you?" "Will you?" "Have you?" or "Are you?" Imagine asking your child:

"Did you try the chicken?"

"Can you please finish your sandwich?"

"Will you take at least one bite?"

"Have you even tasted the stew?"

"Are you eating any beans?"

How would they reply?

Closed-ended questions arrest kids' zest for eating. They're magnets for meltdowns and so pervasive they make up an entire category of old table talk. But don't become dismayed when you try to avoid them, because it's impossible to completely eradicate closed-ended questions. Your goal is to minimize them, not to achieve a zero-sum game.

When you catch yourself asking a closed question, pause even if you're in the middle of the sentence. Then reword what you want to say in the form of an open-ended question. Do this as often as you can. The easiest trick for transforming table talk from a closed- to an open-ended question is to start with the word "how" or "what." So instead of asking "Did you try the kiwi?" say, "What's most interesting about kiwi?" Instead of saying "Can you please use your fork," ask "How's that different with a fork?" or "What utensil works best for this food?"

Stop and compare those last three questions. Do you hear how ditching "can" and starting with "how" or "what" changes the question from closed- to open-ended? You're creating new table talk! It runs on boundless questions that get you and your child out of ruts. At the end of this chapter, you'll find more examples of open-ended new table talk. For now, your goal is to improve your ratio of open- to closed-ended questions. This assures closed quips aren't the main ingredient in your table talk.

The last thing about closed-ended questions is managing guilt when they inevitably slip your lips. If closed-ended questions run rampant in your table talk, be patient with yourself. The more you practice, the more open-ended questions appear naturally in your table talk. Start questions with "how" or "what," and let go of regret about the rest. Remember, new table talk is a continuous practice and not something you perfect. As a reminder of this, I keep a card on my desk given to me by a mentor. It says, "Forgive. Also, yourself."

Why Open-Ended Questions Work Best

Open-ended questions are the crème de la crème of questions, whether your child loves or loathes a food. If your child gobbles broccoli with glee, say, "Tell me what you notice about broccoli." This can elicit rich responses about color, texture, mouth feel, and flavor. When they howl, "I HATE broccoli!" your table talk remains the same. "Tell me what you notice about broccoli" gives even the hater a chance to be heard.

You may be thinking *Hold on. I already know my kid's opinion of broccoli. I just want them to eat a green vegetable every once in a blue moon!* I get it. Parenting how kids eat is hard enough already. If this all sounds like a superfluous stunt you don't have time or energy for, you're not alone. When I first teach my clients about open- versus closed-ended table talk, they often furrow their brow and then ask, "Will changing the kinds of questions I ask make my kid eat better?" The short answer is yes, but the proof is in the pudding. My intent in sharing this method is that you'll test it out for yourself.

There are several ways open-ended questions work better than their closed-ended counterparts, not the least of which is all parents (myself included) often use closed-ended questions inadvertently. Increased consciousness and rewording to any degree is an upgrade. Parents who swap closed-ended questions for the open-ended variety report that even this one change leads to less energy drain at the table. That's because with new table talk you establish a consistent pattern of communication regardless of your child's food whims. Open-ended questions give you confidence, clarity, and something useful to say to your child in the flashpoint of food struggles. Open-ended questions help kids eat better by not entertaining the fight. Your words don't egg kids on but turn them inward to explore their experience.

My clients Carrie and Eric exemplify this. They credit new table talk with changing their family's mealtime climate. There's less fussing and more cooperation during meals with their seven- and twelve-year-old kids. Carrie sought my help because, in her words, she "didn't want to make the kids crazy about food like my parents did with me." The challenges Carrie and Eric face include parenting two very different eaters—reminding one kid to slow down and the other to stay focused during meals. When their oldest child began sneaking and hiding food, it put Carrie and Eric on edge. They knew not to scold but were unsure how to teach their kids to make "good choices" without helicopter parenting around food.

Eric was openly doubtful at first that new table talk could make any difference. Implementing open-ended questions changed his mind. He says, "Open-ended questions calm me down and stop me from second-guessing how I talk to the kids about eating. I hear them out, help where I can, and let go of the rest. It's a relief to not get so tangled up in food battles."

What Carrie appreciates about new table talk is how it stands the test of time. The family started using new table talk five years ago, and Carrie says, "Now that our oldest is a tween, I see even more benefits from having established this way of talking about food. I ask my kids questions about eating that I needed to hear myself!" Carrie and Eric's new table talk has become a spoken family value, bringing more levity to family meals.

Open-ended questions do that sort of thing. They give kids the freedom to relate to food and their experience of eating without old table talk getting in the way. That means kids' exploration of food and eating can unfold instead of being dismissed or overruled. We don't often realize how old table talk brushes off or overrides aspects of kid's eating, which brings us to the next type of question we'll discuss. I call these *prove-it questions*.

Prove-It Questions

Prove-it questions are tricky because they sound open-ended but they operate with undertones that reinforce rigidity about eating. Prove-it questions have a passive-aggressive vibe, even when dressed up in an open-ended disguise. They're the table talk equivalent of the wolf in grandmother's clothing. Parents usually ask prove-it questions when kids resist or reject a food. When kids shout, "I don't like chili!" parents often say, "How do you know? You didn't even taste it!" Or they ask, "What do you mean?" implying *there's nothing wrong with this chili*. Or "What don't you like?"

Reread those three questions. See how they're technically open-ended but dubious and snarly sounding? These are prove-it questions, and they cause one bitter effect: kids dig in their heels to assert their autonomy as eaters.

When a kid thinks a food is gross, whether they've tried it or not, prove-it questions hand them a mic to justify their revulsion. The interchangeable answers to "Why don't you like chili?" or "How do you know if you didn't even try it?!" are "Because" and "I just don't." Now you're stuck in a table talk trap.

Prove-it questions disrupt how kids build self-trust as eaters. They also weaken parent-child dialogue by putting kids, and ultimately parents, on the defensive. There's nothing kids hate more during meals than a parent down their throat about food. Simply put, prove-it questions sour eating situations. They cause kids to feel provoked, which leads to undesirable outcomes for everyone.

The key to doing away with prove-it questions is prioritizing curiosity over consumption. So invite your child to share their observations and experience of "chili" (or food they're rejecting), whatever their thoughts and experience may be. Eliminate expectations to eat. Tap into your child's experience of seeing, smelling, hearing, touching, or imagining something about the food (notice how I left out the word "tasting"). Above all, listen nonjudgmentally to their response. For example, your child might describe things they loathe about chili (noteworthy and valuable), or they might surprise you and make up a story about kidney beans on a pole. Either way, you're not stacking the deck toward aversion. You're opening the door for a gastronomically intelligent eating experience. Kids can feel a difference when you improve your table talk questions. They're on the receiving end of someone listening to their struggle.

Here's some new table talk for when your child rejects food (replace *chili* with whatever food suits your situation):

"What do you notice about chili?"

"I'm hearing you aren't interested in chili right now. That's okay."

"You have a lot to say about chili. I'm listening. How does the chili look [smell, sound, or feel] for you?" (Ask about just one of the senses at a time.)

You can also say "I won't make you eat it," if that's true and it resonates with your food philosophy. If you're sick of saying that or aren't sure what to say after you say that, stay tuned. We'll tackle that scenario in a few pages. For now, let's work on cutting out prove-it questions.

How to Root Out Prove-It Questions

When you find yourself up the prove-it-question creek, you have a decision to make. You can intentionally stop talking (about the food your kid is avoiding) or you can try a new open-ended question, one without an edge. Ask yourself the following questions. They'll help you determine whether to say more or just leave things be.

1. Can you mentally acknowledge your child's basic goodness and vulnerability as an eater *in this moment*? Can you see through whatever behavior they're exhibiting and speak directly to their GI core? If yes, proceed to question two. If no, say nothing.

2. What's your purpose in asking this question? Are you trying to enhance curiosity and connection or are you trying to make your kid eat chili? If your focus is getting curious about chili or connecting with your child in this conundrum, go ahead with an open-ended question. If not, say nothing.

The only other thing to consider is how worked up your child is. If they're on the floor wailing, don't ask more questions. If your child is mild- to medium-level upset (which only you can gauge), say calmly, "It seems like there's trouble with the chili." If they soften to that (even with eye contact), ask empathetically, "What does the chili [feel/smell/look/sound] like for you?" (Choose only one of the senses.) Maybe you gently hold their hand, or offer whatever nonverbal gesture shows them you're right here listening. Your sincere attention—even for a few seconds—can really make a difference. If your child speaks, listen carefully. Don't devalue or disagree with what they say. You're not trying to make them swallow chili (or their pride), even if that's what you've previously done.

You're helping them call upon their gastronomic intelligence, so both of you have something substantive to work with.

Here's an example of how this works in one family. Daphne is two and she won't eat chili. It upsets her beyond words. Despite this, she grabs fresh cilantro, sniffs it, and happily plucks leaves off stems. Intrigued with touching and smelling cilantro, Daphne replies to her dad's new table talk with enthusiasm. He keeps things simple and open-ended: "How's the cilantro feel?" This elicits her devilish grin and gastronomically eloquent reply, "Sorta slimy!" Daphne's dad has learned to omit prove-it questions like "How about you try the chili with some cilantro?" or "What's wrong with chili?" Instead, he uses table talk focusing on one of the five senses. His open-ended questions are less about the food and more about Daphne's experience. That's how you avoid prove-it questions.

Even amongst reluctant eaters, the five senses are doorways to explore all aspects of eating. Using sensory observations as the basis for open-ended questions piques interest and preserves an open-mindedness about food. Daphne is hands-and-nose on, even with foods that aren't her thing. Her parents new table talk matches what naturally compels and keeps her engaged.

But sniffing cilantro doesn't count as a meal, so what happens if Daphne doesn't actually eat dinner? In the early stages of transforming your table talk, it's a matter of sticking with the method, because open, curious, and nonobligatory language helps kids inch closer to eating foods they would otherwise resist. None of this precludes you from serving at least one food you know your child will eat. New table talk still matters, however, because it's how you break the routine when your kid eats a narrow range of foods. A few weeks after Daphne's parents introduced new table talk, she started eating chili, albeit in a deconstructed form. She picks out kidney beans, squeezes fresh lime (add-on), and says, "It's not too *pice-eee!*" (spicy).

We've covered two types of questions to avoid (prove-it and closed-ended) and earmarked open-ended questions as a way forward. The last type of question is called a probing question, and it's desirable too.

Probing Questions

Probing questions are what you ask to get a little more detail about something your child says. Since your role is to elicit and then listen to your child's observations about food and eating, you'll want to take what they say and use it to formulate probing questions. You may not be surprised to hear probing questions work best when they're open-ended.

When your child says crackers or celery are "crunchy," open-ended probing questions to ask include "Where do you feel that crunch?" or "What part of your body senses [or gets] the crunching?" Listen to your child's description without trying to revise or persuade them about anything. If you're getting blank stares, share a comment about where you notice crunchiness (in your ears, teeth, tongue, jaw, for example). Open-ended probing questions do the important work of reminding you to eat with awareness. With very few words, they stoke curiosity in fresh ways. A simple "What else?" is a probing question inviting your child to keep exploring. What else do they notice with this food?

Kids appreciate open-ended probing questions because they give them a special feeling: *You've never asked me this before!* Children are driven by the power of inquiry. With food, that's a gift that keeps on giving. Asking them these questions during meals helps kids feel competent and captivated. *How interesting that my parents want to hear what I think and feel while I eat!* This also teaches kids that their internal experiences around food are worth paying attention to, continuing to reinforce gastronomic intelligence.

The main pitfall of probing questions is when parents start out open-ended but then revert to close-ended questions in follow-up. The dialogue below highlights this problem. It's a short exchange between Barb and her four-year-old son, Henry, who's avoiding his soup. After each of Barb's quotes, I've labeled the type of table talk she's using. Read the conversation twice. First, skip what's in the brackets, and just get the gist of what's being said. Then, go back and notice the types of questions and their impact.

Barb:	My soup is steaming! Henry, what are you noticing?
	[comment from her own experience + open-ended question]
Henry:	I don't want soup.
Barb:	Did you try it? [closed-ended question]
Henry:	No.
Barb:	Can you try just one bite, please? [closed-ended question]
Henry:	I don't want to.

Barb led with a comment based on her own experience plus an open-ended question but slid back into closed-question mode after that. Her closed-ended probing questions fail to intrigue, engage, or empower Henry in terms of his soup. The method for avoiding the pitfall of closed-ended questions is to use reflective statements instead.

Reflective Statements

Reflective statements aren't questions but fruitful phrases that summarize what your child is observing or implying about food or eating. Reflective statements in the Table Talk Method often begin with three magic words: "It seems like…" or "It sounds like…" Use either of these sentence starters and finish them off with a paraphrased version of whatever your child says or feels about the food. For example, when your child says, "I don't want beets," you reply, "It sounds like you're not into the beets." It might seem absurd to parrot back your kid's comment, but this is a crucial pivot point. Reflective statements tell your child they're being heard. That simple acknowledgment leads you down a different path, away from bickering or serving separate meals. Reflective statements get kids consulting their gastronomic intelligence. And that's just the beginning of how reflective statements work.

Let's revisit the same soup scenario between Barb and Henry. This time notice how Barb skillfully replaces closed-ended probing questions with reflective statements and how that changes the interaction.

Barb: My soup is steaming! Henry, what are you noticing? [comment from her own experience + open-ended question]

Henry: I don't want soup.

Barb: It sounds like soup isn't interesting you right now. [reflective statement]

Henry: Yah, I'm not in the mood for soup.

Barb: What are you noticing about the soup? [open-ended question]

Henry: (*Sadly resting his chin in one hand.*) It's tomatoey...and too lumpy.

Barb: So it feels lumpy for you. What would help it? [reflective statement + open-ended question]

Can you hear how Barb's use of reflective statements and open-ended questions acknowledge the upset vibe of this meal? Barb gives Henry space for disappointment without getting him different food. Soup's on the table, and it doesn't have to ruin everything. Barb's reflective statements tell Henry she's listening. He feels heard and doesn't resort to additional defense mechanisms to dodge the soup.

Barb asking Henry to share what the soup is like for him softens the stalemate over soup, creating a bit of wiggle room. What was a hard stop ("I don't want soup") shifts ever so slightly to reveal a sliver of possibility. That's the narrow margin you work with when managing food struggles, which makes it easy to see why things often just devolve into a meltdown. New table talk doesn't make Henry dive into that soup, but it sparks the chance for less conflict.

Henry doesn't feel like eating the soup. No surprise there. Yet he shows his GI chops by using two adjectives, "tomatoey" and "lumpy." Barb triggers this type of intuiting by using reflective statements. Her new table talk gets Henry linked up with his inner awareness of eating. In terms of healthy eating habits, that's way more important than whether or not he eats this soup!

Reflective statements encourage self-discovery, self-trust, and greater flexibility around food. Each of these things are an exit ramp when kids break down over food. Henry being invited to say what's going on with the soup gives him more than just a sense of control. The license to describe his felt sense of soup provides new options for both Henry and Barb. First, it makes available a potential work-around rooted in Henry's own gastronomic intelligence (the add-on). Second, it releases Barb from a hard-and-fast storyline about Henry's stubbornness with soup. Without Barb's reflective statements, both possibilities would be missed.

The add-on method (taught in chapter 5) resolves this struggle by helping kids live with food that isn't hoped for or preferred. It's Henry stomaching that lumpy soup with something added-on if he chooses. That's another thing reflective statements do for you. They liberate you from being a short-order cook! Barb's reflective statement paired with an open-ended question shows she has registered Henry's observations (in this case, grievances) and is entrusting him to figure out how to handle the situation. Barb asking "What would help it?" gives Henry the power to modify and make do with the soup before him. It also prevents Barb from succumbing to old table talk like "This is what's for dinner, so just eat it" or "You can eat it now, or you can eat it later."

Reflective statements serve four purposes in the Table Talk Method:

- They demonstrate parents are truly listening, trying to connect with their child, and trying to understand their moment-to-moment experiences of food and process of eating.

- They orient kids to their inner experiences of eating, teaching them to recognize and value those observations.

- They prevent parents from backsliding into old table talk, by cueing more open-ended questions.

- They uphold gastronomic intelligence (self-trust, self-satisfaction, and self-compassion around eating).

Reflective statements are one of the most powerful ways parents can affirm kids' sovereignty as eaters. In *The Awakened Family*, Shefali Tsabary describes what children need to truly thrive: "They need us to mirror back to them how rich they are in their capacity for accomplishment and ability to run their own life" (2017, 32). Reflective statements are a key component of new table talk, because they succinctly convey a sense of adequacy and agency for kids, not based on how well they are (or aren't) performing as an eater.

Reflective statements paired with open-ended questions are a great alternative to old table talk. They make an especially useful combination to replace conditional table talk. Reflective statements paired with open-ended questions provide kids with a radical takeaway: *Deep down, my parents believe in my ability to manage my own eating.* Sadly, this sentiment isn't often reflected in how we speak to kids while they eat, even when it's truly what we intend to convey. Adopting new table talk that acknowledges kids' competence and capability with food and eating is critical and very different from the message kids habitually receive from old table talk ways.

By now we've covered all five communication skills, so let's review. When creating new table talk, your goal is to use open-ended questions, probing questions, and reflective statements as often as you can while limiting closed-ended and prove-it questions. A simple way to frame this is to wonder with your child about eating more than you worry about how they eat. The best thing you can do to raise happy, healthy eaters is to partner with your kids in exploratory eating with new table talk.

Practicing New Table Talk

You've got the basics of the Table Talk Method down: bring curiosity, connection, five senses–based eating, and adjectives to mealtimes with your child to nurture gastronomic intelligence. You also have the pieces you need to create new table talk phrases. You're already using new language like "What do you notice?" "Tell me about," "It seems like," and "What would help it?" This next section offers a new table talk buffet to add on to what you've already learned.

The new table talk phrases listed here replace old table talk. If the examples sound odd, that's to be expected. Adjusting what you say to your child about eating is a novel approach, and changing your words to manage food conflict is a far cry from how things usually get done. Asking "What do you notice about onions?" might sound strange at first. Pay close attention, however, to how your child responds and how new table talk affects your own state-of-being. What basic things happen at the table when you use open-ended questions and reflective statements? What's the general vibe of your meals now that you're using new table talk?

Use New Table Talk Phrases

These questions and sentence starters are new table talk options to choose from. You'll find open-ended questions, probing questions, and reflective statements, which you can adapt and bring to your family table.

Two core phrases:

- "What do you notice?"

- "Tell me about..."

Start questions with "how..." or "what...":

- "What would help it?"

- "How's the zucchini, for you?"

- "What flavors do you notice?"

- "How's the pineapple tasting?"

- "What's the plan for your chili?"

- "How [or where] are you going to start?"

- "What's your next bite? I'm trying to guess..."

Anchor inquiries to one of the five senses:

- "What do you notice about how raisins look?"

- "Using smelling [leaning forward to demonstrate], what's your nose getting from this waffle?"

- "How's the cauliflower feel on your tongue?" or "What's your tongue noticing?"

- "What flavor [or smell] are you picking up on?"

- "Tell me about the texture of edamame, for you."

- "What's it like feeling kiwi?"

- "What do you notice touching this salad?"

- "What's the sound of pistachios?"

- "How does asparagus look twirling?"

- "How do black beans feel, mashed?"

- "I'm interested to see how this piece looks with that bite!"

- "I'm wondering what you notice?" Refer to touch, sight, smell, flavor, or sound.

Start with the words "I'm curious...":

- "I'm curious, what happens when you squish a grape?"

- "I'm curious about the color inside a blueberry?"

- "I'm curious if this beet can stamp a print on my plate?"

- "I'm curious to hear what you notice about the stew?"

- "I'm curious about how that bite sounds to you?"

- "I'm curious, how does that bite smell [look, taste, or feel]?"

- "I'm curious what you'll choose for your first bite?" Or "Your next bite?" "Your last bite?"

Practice reflective statements:

- "It seems like..."

- "It sounds like..."

- "I remember you said..."

- "You were saying..."

- "That's interesting..."

This chart gives a variety of responses to your kid in different situations. The middle column shows language you're trying to leave behind, and the column on the right offers new table talk to replace it. Use this chart to help transform your table talk from old to new. Adapt these lines to whatever food applies. This chart is also available at http://www .newharbinger.com/49463.

Say This Instead

When your kid says:	Don't say (old table talk):	Try this (new table talk):
"I don't want salmon."	"You didn't even try it yet. This time might be different." "Take a no-thank-you bite. If you still don't want it, you don't have to eat it."	"What are you noticing about the salmon?" "What's making salmon hard to see [smell/touch/ taste] right now?" "What would help it?"
"I don't like peppers."	"Try a little to be sure." "Did you try it? You can't say you don't like it until you've tried it." "Why don't you try a bite? You might like it."	"Tell me about peppers." "I'm curious how these peppers look [smell/feel] for you?" "It sounds like peppers feel…" "What would help them?"
"Get the tofu off my plate! Yuck!"	"You can't just have rice. You need to eat some protein too." "Just leave it on the side of your plate."	"It seems like there's trouble with the tofu. What do you notice about it?" "What's this tofu like for you?" "What would help it?"

"I'm not eating stir-fry."	"You don't have to like it, but you do have to try it."	"How do you feel seeing [smelling/tasting/touching] stir-fry?" "What are you noticing about stir-fry?"
"Why can't I have more chips?"	"I'm sorry, no more chips." "You can't just eat chips."	"Chips aren't part of dinner tonight." "How we can bring part of what you love about chips (crunch, salt) to the food for dinner tonight?"
"Why do we *always* have to eat salad?"	"Last time you ate salad, you liked it!" "What don't you like about salad?"	"It sounds like you're not in the mood for salad." "Tell me about the smell [sight/sound] of salad for you." "What parts [things] do you notice in this salad?"
"I'm done." (They barely touched their plate).	"Did you eat any beans?" "How much rice did you have?" "You didn't eat enough." "Please eat now, so you're not hungry later."	"What's the plan for your beans?" "How can we use that later?" "Which unused food should we save [keep] fresh?" "Where's the full feeling in your body?"

With a full menu of new table talk at your disposal, let's see how it's sinking in. The next short quiz tests your knowledge of new table talk.

EXERCISE: New Table Talk Quiz

Circle the new table talk reply for each kid quote or behavior below. (Hint: Look for open-ended questions, probing questions, and reflective statements.) An answer key appears at the end of this chapter.

1. "I don't like brussels sprouts."

    a. "What don't you like?"

    b. "You liked them last time we had them."

    c. "Why don't you like them?"

    d. "How about you try one bite and see?"

    e. "What would help them?"

2. "Oh, *come on*, do we have to have meatloaf?! We ate that last week!"

    a. "We didn't have it last week, and yes, it's what's for dinner."

    b. "I'm sorry you don't want meatloaf, but that's what we're having."

    c. "Tell me what you notice about meatloaf."

    d. "You're not getting a separate meal."

    e. "Taste buds change all the time, so who knows? You might like it tonight."

3. "But I *hate* salmon!"

    a. "You should hear what it says about you!"

    b. "You didn't try this kind yet."

    c. "Is there something else on the table you'd like more of?"

    d. "What's the salmon like for you?"

    e. "You used to like it! This is the same recipe as always."

4. "Can we get ice cream? Please? *Puh-lease* can we get ice cream? Why can't we get ice cream?" (Repeat.)

   a. "It sounds like you're in the mood for something smooth and sweet!"

   b. "If you get your homework done, we can talk about it."

   c. "You've had too much ice cream lately."

   d. "Didn't you just have ice cream at Josie's house?"

   e. "Maybe if you eat a good lunch."

5. Child avoiding a food on the plate. For example, cabbage is entirely untouched.

   a. "Do you like the cabbage?"

   b. "Will you please just try the cabbage?"

   c. "Take two bites of cabbage, then you can be done."

   d. "Where does cabbage live when it's growing up?"

   e. "What do you have against cabbage?"

You've investigated your old table talk tendencies and separated from those words. They were honest attempts to get your kids eating well, but they didn't produce the desired results. You understand the counterproductive nature of old table talk and have a whole new set of skills to use. The best tools for constructing new table talk are open-ended questions, probing questions, and reflective statements. In the next chapter, we'll add one more skill (ING-verbs) and consolidate what you've learned about language into three formulas. You'll keep advancing your table talk repertoire and mix and match things to suit your needs.

Quiz answers: 1.e, 2.c, 3.d, 4.a, 5.d

CHAPTER 7

Apply New Table Talk Formulas for Success

Lorna was pressured to eat as a child because of her small stature. Now as a mother of two, she avoids saying things to her kids about eating for fear her words will make them feel like she did growing up. When her four-year-old rejects food, Lorna suppresses table talk, swallowing her words in a conflicted effort not to impose. She desperately wants to have a positive influence on how and what her kids eat but feels uncertain what to say to safeguard their sovereignty as eaters. How does new table talk encourage kids to eat without pressuring them? What can you say to correct bad manners or appreciate kids trying new things? And how do you coach technicalities of eating without using old table talk?

New table talk can be organized into three basic formulas. They're the blueprints you'll get in this chapter to consistently generate new table talk that nurtures gastronomic intelligence. Your exact words will vary based on what your child says and does at the table, but you'll have the basic recipes to respond with mindful awareness and new table talk, time and again.

The structure of these formulas supports your long-term use of new table talk, meaning as your child ages and food challenges take on new themes, you'll still have reliable communication tools. The formulas teach you to use reflective statements instead of conditional table talk and to trade out words that expect and oblige with words that promote more mindful eating. They show you how to praise and appreciate your child's eating not solely by acknowledging the deed but by asking them a self-reflective question. They also tell you what to say when you want to instruct or correct something about your child's eating.

New Table Talk Formulas

The three new table talk formulas offered here are based on skills you've already learned. What follows are instructions for using each formula along with plenty of examples. These formulas aren't prescriptive, in the sense that you must stick to the script. They provide a framework for you to create new table talk that feels and sounds natural to you.

Formula One = Open-Ended Question

Formula one is you asking an open-ended question. That's the mainstay of your new table talk. It's a reliable method you can use anytime to undo expectations around eating and alleviate obligatory stuff (like the try-bite). Open-ended questions are also essential additions to the end of any comments you make appreciating or praising how your child eats.

To use this formula, sit down to eat with your child. Pick one of the five senses that naturally pique your interest based on the food in front of you. Guide your child's exploration of sight, smell, touch, flavor, or sound by asking an open-ended question. Don't make this a big production. Don't announce, "We're going to try a new way of eating!" Simply ask an open-ended question like "How's your green veggie tonight?" or "How do the carrots smell?" Then listen—attentively—to what your child has to say. Dig deeper with probing questions that also maintain an open-ended format. Elicit your child's experience of eating with open-ended questions that prompt them to tune in, again and again, to seeing, smelling, chewing, feeling, and hearing while they eat.

Here are some examples of formula one:

"Which taste does your tongue want first [or next]?"

"What's your first bite going to be?"

"How's that feel on your tongue?"

Formula Two = Reflective Statement + Open-Ended Question

Formula two is a reflective statement plus an open-ended question. As a reminder reflective statements start in one of two ways: either with these three magic words ("It seems like" or "It sounds like") or with you sharing an observation from your own eating. Whichever option you start with, add an open-ended question to the end, so your reflective statement is paired with an open-ended question. This formula corrects conditional table talk (if-then eating), and it's also the best way to praise or appreciate your child trying new foods. Two versions of this formula are broken down below.

OPTION ONE = THREE MAGIC WORDS + OPEN-ENDED QUESTION

This is when you paraphrase something your child says or feels about food, starting with "It sounds like" or "It seems like" and follow up with an open-ended question. Examples of this option are:

"It sounds like mushrooms aren't doing it for you. I'm curious what you see [smell, feel, or hear]?"

"It seems like the mac and cheese is spot-on for you tonight. What do you notice?

OPTION TWO = YOUR SENSORY OBSERVATION + OPEN-ENDED QUESTION

This is where you lead with your own noticing. Describe what's going on with one of your five senses and the food you're eating. Pick one or two adjectives and offer your observation. Keep your comment brief, and follow up with an open-ended question, so it comes together like this: "These blueberries really pop. For me, they're tart and juicy. How about for you?" Don't say anything about what you want your child to notice, feel, or eat. After you share your adjectives, ask your child what they notice. Be their curious companion exploring your own senses while skillfully asking about theirs. One quick reminder about which type of adjectives to use: avoid words that label food as good or bad. Choose words that describe what your senses detect—things like smooth, creamy, or crunchy.

Here are some examples:

"For me, this is crisp. What do you notice?"

"I'm noticing smoothness. What do you see [or feel, taste, smell, or hear]?"

"This sauce tastes tangy to me. What's the flavor for you?"

"This sorbet feels cold and silky in my mouth. What's the feeling for you?"

"I'm smelling [lean forward, sniffing food]…cinnamon. How about you?"

Formula Three = ING-Verb

Formula three features one ING-verb as the first (or only) word of new table talk. Use this formula when you feel the urge to change something about your child's eating. ING-verbs were introduced in chapter 1 (with the perennial theme of kids wiping food on their clothes), but this formula works for many displeasing habits, like kids talking with a mouthful of food or eating off of or using your plate as a dumping ground.

The ING-formula has two versions. Both versions done compassionately work to oust shame inherent in old table talk.

OPTION ONE = ING-VERB (YOU MIME THE ACTION)

The first option is to say just one word, the ING-tense of the action you want your child to take, while you demonstrate it. Here are some examples of how to do this:

When kids wipe hands or face on clothes, say "Wiping." (Simultaneously wipe your hands on your napkin without any extra comments.)

When kids can't stay put in their chair, say "Sitting." (Wiggle your own seat a bit to show where you butt meets the chair).

When kids are talking while chewing, you say "Chewing." (Show chewing with your lips closed. If that doesn't work, you can put a finger to your lips to gesture *no talking*, but do this only as a last resort.)

When kids talk with their mouth full of food, say "Closing." (Open, then seal your lips.)

When kids pick apart or rip tiny pieces off a bagel or a sandwich, say "Biting." (Demonstrate biting into that food.)

When crumbs or dribbles of food are going all over the place, and you want your child to eat over their plate, say, "Leaning." (Demonstrate leaning forward over your own plate.)

OPTION TWO = ING-VERB + GENTLE SUGGESTION

The second way to use an ING-verb is offering a kind suggestion. Use this option to lend a hand when your child starts getting worked up about eating or shows signs of uneasiness with food. This might sound like instructive table talk, but the difference is you're emphasizing the new action rather than spotlighting faults or manners that need "correcting." Your words present an option for your child, not an old table talk command. The tone must be empathetic and hospitable, soothing not stern. The unspoken sentiment is *It's okay to feel this. I see your struggle, and I want to help.* You're showing your child that you get it. Strong feelings come up when we eat—even for adults! It's nothing to feel bad about, but it is something kids need to learn how to work through. ING-verbs can help.

Here are some examples:

- When kids pick apart food and pile it up (or throw it across the room), say "Leaving those bits here" or "Moving that to the side."

- If you want kids to stop eating off your plate, say "Eating from here." (Rest your hand, palm down next to their plate.)

- When kids want more of a food but still have plenty of uneaten stuff on their plate, say "Working with what's on your plate."

- When kids beg for something other than what's for dinner say, "Choosing from what's on the table."

- If they're not eating much, try "Imagining what flavor [smell, sound, or feeling] might come from that?"

Finally, if you think your child is overeating, don't comment to that effect. Say nothing about "giving it a few minutes," "slowing down," or "holding back." It's true, those are all ING-verbs, but they encroach on your child's responsibilities as an eater to decide if and how much they'll eat from what's served. When you feel the need to direct or correct something about your child's eating, choose ING-verbs that honor Satter's division of responsibility in feeding. In chapter 8, you'll learn some new ways to ask your child about hunger and fullness.

With any and all new table talk, how you say things is important. The nonverbal tone you're going for is like a highly effective yoga instructor, cueing with clarity and warmth, not overcoaching or giving orders. You want your voice and body language to nudge your kid in the right direction, not bog them down with audible sighs or sidelong glances. New table talk should feel not like you're calling kids out but like you're gently guiding them inward.

Finding Your New Table Talk Stride

Now that you're familiar with new table talk, which formulas feel most natural to you? Play around with all the options in a variety of situations to figure out what works best. If it's hard to know which formula to use, consult the quick fixes chart coming up next. It shows the simplest way to undo each type of old table talk. You can also try any open-ended question and see where it takes you. Sampling all kinds of new table talk will help you find your favorites. Remember to use this framework in good as well as bad times—these words aren't only meant for meltdowns!

With ongoing practice, you will reach a point where you don't think about new table talk as formulaic. You'll ask open-ended questions and use reflective statements and ING-verbs fluently. That takes time, however, and for some families it involves growing pains because parents and kids have gotten used to how old table talk ruled the roost. The six-year-old child of one family ate up her parents' new table talk, but in the first few days kept asking them "So how many bites do I have to eat before I get dessert?"

Table talk, at least some of the old stuff, might have established rules and regulations around food. So when you transition to open-ended questions and ditch conditional and obligatory language, it may take a few days for your child to catch on to this new way of doing things. If unplugging old table talk causes operational issues during your family meals, use new table talk. For example, if your child is used to you telling them when they've eaten enough, say, "I trust you to decide how much your body needs." Then add probing questions as needed, like "How full are you feeling right now?" or "Where's the full feeling in your body?" It's never too soon or too late to begin using new table talk like this, because children are gastronomically intelligent beings. Your new words affirm that.

The next chart gives specific suggestions for how to use new table talk formulas to undo patterns of old table talk. The left-hand column lists the main types of old table talk. Locate the type of table talk you want to undo and next to it, in the right-hand column, find the new table talk formula that might have the most impact for you. You're not locked into using one formula or another, but the chart spells out efficient methods to resolve any old table talk still hanging around. This chart is also available at http://www.newharbinger.com/49463.

Quick Fixes for Transforming Old Table Talk

If your old table talk is:	Try this new table talk formula instead:
Instructive: "Lean over your plate, please."	ING-verb: "Leaning." (Demonstrate without extra words.)
Corrective: "Don't chew with your mouth open."	ING-verb: "Closing." (Open, then seal your lips.)
Praise: "Great job trying new things!"	Reflective statement + open-ended question: "It seems like you're really enjoying the hummus. What are you noticing?"
Conditional: "Eat two bites of soup, and then you can have more bread."	Reflective statement + open-ended question: "It seems like the bread is really calling to you. How's it work with the soup?" or "Tell me about the soup for you."
Obligatory: "You don't have to like it, but you do have to try it."	Open-ended question: "What would help it?"
Expectant: "I made this just how you like!"	Open-ended question: "How's this look [smell, feel, or sound] working for you?"
Appreciative: "Thank you for trying your vegetables."	Open-ended question : "How's the color [or smell or texture] of the vegetables for you?"
Closed-ended question: "Do you like the sweet potatoes?"	Open-ended question: "How are the sweet potatoes?"

Bear in mind that you don't have to memorize phrases for every variation of new table talk, and you don't need to preselect your lines. It's all about being present with what's right in front of you. Ask, reflect, or use an ING-verb, and you're using the Table Talk Method. It's a practice—an everyday kind of practice—which means you've got plenty of time, like every meal and snack your child eats between now and when they move out.

If family meals don't happen as often as you'd like, every time your child eats is a chance to relate differently, and new table talk isn't confined to your table. It works on the fly with any and every food encounter, like takeout, picnics, or the ice cream truck. Sometimes it's fun and other times it's frenzied, but both have equal value in terms of table talk learning.

When you're frustrated, remember what helps most is an open-ended question. Ask something about the five senses and the food causing the kerfuffle. Then turn your child's reply into a reflective statement. You're using new table talk and proclaiming more flexibility in how you parent around food! Now that you're rolling with new table talk, jot down your new phrases in your journal. The next exercise gets you adding to the list you already started.

EXERCISE: Add Your New Table Talk

Open your journal to the page titled "My New Table Talk," because you have more to say. Write down the new table talk you've been using lately, and keep adding to the list over the next few days. Maybe your words closely mirror the formulas in this chapter, and maybe some things still sound old-school. Write it all down without judging yourself. What's working will be your inspiration, and what's not is easier to change when you see it written on a page. You'll use this list at the end of this chapter, so don't skip this exercise. Any amount of new table talk you capture will allow you to see results.

You won't be writing table talk down forever, but for now it helps things sink in. It's kind of like overhearing other people's table talk. I edited this chapter at the beach in earshot of a father saying "Sam, you need to eat something now, or you're going to become a crazy person."

Sam's mom tried to help too by adding "It's just chicken tenders. They taste just like the dinosaur ones." Sam spent twenty minutes on his towel and managed three nibbles of chicken. I don't know Sam or his parents, but their lunch made me want to both laugh and cry—I knew so well that feeling as a parent where you just want food to get into your child so you can move on from this meal. But as things came to a head, it was crystal clear that typical, old table talk was unproductive for everyone. Sam picked up his pail and headed back down to the water while his parents kept giving it a go: "Why don't you have more chicken? You need to eat more, Sam. If you don't, we're all going to be sorry!" Every example of table talk you hear is a learning opportunity—whether old or new! And since nothing says it better than real-life examples, let's dissect another true story.

Ninja Noshing with Old Table Talk

In this example, seven-year-old Noelle would rather play Ninja than eat dinner. She shows up at the table, scarfs three bites of pasta, and runs off to play, again and again. This triggers an old table talk exchange:

Dad: Noelle, get back here and eat. You're not getting dessert if you don't eat dinner first.

Noelle: (*Traipsing back to the table, eats one noodle while standing up.*)

Dad: Sit down NOW. Please. And eat your dinner.

Noelle: (*Scowls, sits down, and starts pushing food around on her plate.*) I don't want salad.

Dad: You need to eat some vegetables. Just take two bites.

Noelle: I don't like salad.

Dad: You didn't even try it!

Noelle: It's gross. Can I have more pasta?"

Mom:	You had this *same salad* last week and loved it.
Noelle:	But I don't want it. I want more pasta.
Dad:	You can't just eat pasta, Noelle. You need to have some salad too.
Noelle:	I'm all done.
Dad:	Well…okay, but salad is what you're getting when you say you're hungry later.
Noelle:	(*Stuffs two forkfuls of pasta into her mouth and leaves the table in a huff.*)
Mom:	Noelle, did you eat enough? (*Sigh.*) Please get back here and eat some dinner.
Noelle:	(*Ignores the request.*)
Dad:	That's it, Noelle, you're not getting cookies tonight.

What do you notice about the table talk Noelle's parents employ? How effective is their approach at engaging Noelle with dinner? This wrenchingly familiar back-and-forth contains a hodgepodge of old table talk. There are instructive, conditional, and expectant utterances, none of which prove productive. Noelle's parents ask her only one question. Did you spot it? It's the closed-ended "Did you eat enough?" Unsurprisingly, this question garners no response.

What's missing from this mealtime scene is new table talk rooted in curiosity and connection. Open-ended questions, ING-verbs, and reflective statements are what Noelle needs to "focus on eating" by accessing her gastronomic intelligence. Noelle's distractibility at dinner has less to do with salad than with the talk at the table. Sure, she likes one food (pasta) and not the other (salad), and she'd much rather be playing. But doesn't that describe how most first graders eat?

The problem is the lack of language that would help Noelle get in touch with her body or senses as an eater. All that's available is old table talk. No questions about what Noelle is noticing, feeling, or experiencing with hunger or the food. Any of the new table talk formulas you've learned could improve this situation in terms of Noelle's engagement with food and her parent's frustration. You've got ideas for how to deal with this now. How would you rewrite the table talk in this story to express curiosity and connection? How could Noelle's parents respond differently?

Ninja Noshing with New Table Talk

Below is a revised dialogue between Noelle and her parents using new table talk. We'll pick it up where the brouhaha began.

Dad: Coming back to the table, Noelle. It's time to eat.

Noelle: (*Traipsing back to the table, eats one noodle while standing up.*)

Dad: Sitting. (*Wiggles in his seat to show where his bottom meets the chair.*)

Noelle: (*Scowls, sits down, and starts pushing food around on her plate.*) I don't want salad.

Dad: What are you noticing about the salad?

Noelle: I don't like it.

Dad: Which part?

Noelle: All of it.

Dad: How's the salad smell for you?

Noelle: It's too sour. (*Noelle doesn't actually smell or taste the salad, but Dad intentionally ignores that.*)

Dad: So you're noticing sour…What else?

Noelle: Um. (*Looking annoyed.*) It's green and wet.

Dad:	I wonder how wet green salad sounds? (*Loads his own fork with salad, unceremoniously.*)
Noelle:	It's gonna sound wimpy.
Dad:	(*Grins.*) Wimpy. What do Ninja's eat to power up?
Noelle:	(*Stuffs two more forkfuls of pasta into her mouth but stays at the table.*) I'm still hungry but not for salad. I want something else.
Mom:	Salad and pasta are what's for dinner. What would help it?

Let's compare the two versions of this story. The original interaction had zero open-ended questions, reflective statements, or ING-verbs. The new table talk version includes all three from the Table Talk Method. I count seven open-ended questions, one reflective statement, and two ING-verbs. Version two has fewer words and is less hassle for everyone. Noelle's not enthusiastic about salad, but she manages to stay more engaged because her parents new table talk invites curiosity and connection. Noelle uses adjectives like *wet* and *green* to process her sense of salad instead of griping and thinking up generic objections. But does Noelle actually eat any salad? Is her plate saved for later? Does this ninja go to bed hungry? *Yes* might be the answer to any or all of these questions depending on a host of factors, many of which aren't in her parents' control. The one thing you have as an ever-present option is your responsiveness with new table talk. It won't make family meals all unicorns and rainbows, but practiced consistently, new table talk shifts how and what your child eats.

When you serve up open-ended questions, reflective statements, and ING-verbs, you might find that your child is paying attention to eating in ways you didn't realize or give them enough credit for. With different questions, you'll get to know how foods feel for your child. They might even get mildly curious about foods they've never had before. Maybe they're sorting out what hums and what doesn't for them with a food? There's tremendous value in encouraging their curiosity, for more than just meltdown prevention.

Noelle's parents' new table talk keeps them out of the red zone with food struggles. How they speak to her about her eating while she's eating empowers her to access her gastronomic intelligence. That's a difference she can feel. It's a lot less agitating to eat when the table talk you absorb welcomes you to your own body. That's how the Table Talk Method differs from other perspectives on feeding kids. Getting Noelle to *want* to eat salad, to *choose* and *enjoy* eating salad, involves more than repeatedly putting small portions on her plate. Veggie exposure just means Noelle is in the vicinity of salad. Proximity alone doesn't move the needle to get your child eating well. It's what you do and say in those moments of nearness that makes all the difference.

Eating is an intimate, sensory-rich process begging for our increased awareness. Kids don't need us to tell them that. They need us to speak to them about their eating in a way that honors this fact. New table talk is about small freedoms you and your child gain when you coach how and what they eat with mindful awareness and effective communication.

How Can You Tell If It's Working?

Progress in the Table Talk Method isn't measured by how many new foods your kid eats or how many meltdowns they have in a certain time period. It's based on skills you see your child exhibit while eating. It's also about your stress level and confidence as you parent your child around food. Sometimes you'll run out of steam and not feel curious or connected at all. That doesn't mean you're failing at this method, at this meal, or with this kid! Any amount of new table talk helps, so don't pressure yourself to achieve some threshold level. It's quality over quantity when it comes to new words. Do your best to stay in the moment and speak from and to what's right in front of you. And keep track of new table talk that feels on point with what you want to teach your child about food and eating.

Self-Reflection Journaling

Turn back in your journal to find your original table talk inventory. This was the list of quotes you gathered in chapter 2. Keep one finger on this page as you turn to your latest journal entries under "My New Table Talk." (If you don't have much on this list yet, you can use your answers from the "Practice New Table Talk" exercise in chapter 5 or return to this self-reflection journaling after you've added new table talk.) Flip back and forth comparing your new words with what you used to say. Take a closer look at your new table talk. Are there open-ended questions, reflective statements, and ING-verbs? With this new language in mind, answer the following questions in your journal.

- How is your new table talk changing things?

- Which specific phrases boost curiosity and connection (between you and your child or your child and their food)?

- When your child complains about food, what do you say? How does it compare to what you said in the past?

- What happens when you use new table talk to address food resistance or rejection? (Example: "What would help it?")

- Which new table talk lowers your stress level during meals?

Over time, most parents find that using new table talk brings more peace and satisfaction during meals and greater appreciation of the inner qualities each family member has as an eater. Discovering these truths on your own through practice can diffuse a lot of tension around food.

New table talk helps you and your child come together over food like you do over books. In chapter 1, I compared eating with reading, at least in how we might teach kids these skills. Old table talk is the equivalent of someone critiquing your experience while you're reading—not just your pronunciation or fluency but how you think and feel on the inside as you relate to the story. When you're reading a book, it doesn't matter what anyone else thinks about that experience. It's happening on an internal landscape—one that's yours to enjoy! We don't try to change or fix that experience for kids when they read. We want them to feel nourished and partake of the joy for themselves. New table talk encourages this in kids of all ages while they eat.

A dear friend asked me about introducing new table talk with her twelve-year-old. She said, "We've been through twelve years of life together. I can't go back in time. And I don't get how asking 'Where's the hungry feeling in your body?' will do much when what they want is another cookie." I welcome her uncertainty because it gets at the heart of why we bother implementing new table talk anyway. You can't predict how your child will respond, and maybe they'll just roll their eyes, but what you put into words with new table talk matters more than calories or nutrients. Your new table talk says, *When it comes to food, stay true to your innermost needs.*

That's a talk I don't hear many parents having with their kids about eating. Sure, new table talk sounds wonky to teens, but so does a lot of other stuff you say. "Can I have another cookie?" isn't a question they'll be asking you much longer, but your (potentially awkward) new table talk helps them gain skills needed to answer that question for themselves.

The three formulas in the Table Talk Method give you the structure to build better phrases. And better phrases prompt healthier behaviors for eaters of all ages. The more you practice, the more often new table talk will show up naturally during meals, with the litmus test being how this new language guides you through the most mundane eating struggles. The next chapter will walk you through some of those everyday eating issues and advance your new table talk to the next level.

CHAPTER 8

Resolve Everyday Eating Dilemmas

Now that you have the foundation and formulas for new table talk, we'll hone your skills by adding to what you've already developed. This will keep you moving in the right direction and reaffirm the heart of the Table Talk Method: to care for struggles around food instead of toiling to make them stop. In this chapter you'll make three final table talk adjustments:

1. Avoid the word "why" when asking a question.

2. Remove the word "too" when you hear your kid say it.

3. Drop these four-letter-words of feeding: "just," "need," "some," and "much."

We'll unpack each of these adjustments in the context of everyday eating dilemmas. You'll learn what to say when kids skip "healthy stuff," when they pick apart what's being served, when they claim they're full (but barely ate a thing), and when they're hungry again ten minutes later. The most important takeaway from this chapter is how to talk with your child about hunger and fullness. I'll also teach you how to eliminate the try-bite if that's something you want to pursue. We could illustrate these final techniques with any number of examples, so don't worry if the challenges you face don't appear here. The techniques in this chapter work across many situations.

Why You Shouldn't Ask Why

The first change in this chapter is getting rid of the word "why," especially when it's the first word you say in a table talk phrase. When your child says, "I hate peppers!" don't ask why, because it's a prove-it question, and prove-it questions amplify conflict around eating (see chapter 6). They prompt kids to defend their behavior or opinion, diverting precious energy to justify why they don't like or want a certain food. So when you catch yourself asking or about to ask this question, pause immediately. Then rephrase what you're saying, so it starts with one of these words instead: "how," "what," "which," "when," or "where." Instead of asking "Why don't you like peppers?" say "Which part of peppers are strongest for you?" or "How do peppers feel [or smell]?"

To get a better understanding of why "Why?" fails, let's consider a complaint I hear often from parents: "My kid doesn't eat the healthy food I pack in their lunch."

The Untouched School Lunch

When food boomerangs back home in your child's lunch box, don't ask, "Why didn't you eat your lunch?" There are only two answers to that question. "I didn't like it" and "I didn't have time." Both might be true, and you've painted yourself into an old table talk corner. "Why" doesn't work because it sets up a you-versus-them inflexibility around food. Remember how prove-it questions arise from a lack of connectedness? Asking your child *why* they're not eating something suggests you're not on their side with eating.

The word "why" also blocks your child's intrinsic curiosity about food. It turns their attention to validating their actions, decisions, and autonomy as an eater. That's a lousy way to feel about eating, whether you're a kid or an adult. Table talk starting with this word puts your child on the spot to deliver an excuse instead of helping them explore new ways of dealing with the problem. "Why" feeds combativeness over food and spoils your child's chance to work with gastronomic intelligence. So next time you find a rank sandwich and slimy produce in their lunch box...

Don't use old table talk:

"Why didn't you eat your lunch?"

"Why didn't you finish your carrots?"

"You said you wanted a turkey-and-cheese wrap. Why'd you leave that behind?"

"You didn't even touch this!" (thinking and maybe saying, "Why do I even bother?")

"Why do you eat the chips and yogurt but nothing else?"

Can you hear how "why" asserts wrongdoing? It's got a divisive feel. Avoid that language by using new table talk suggestions below. These phrases engage your child in collaborative problem solving with open-ended questions and reflective statements, which helps you waste less time, energy, and food.

Use new table talk:

"How can we improve the sandwich [or other food] in your lunch, so it's more satisfying?"

"Which green foods work best at lunch?" or "Which vegetables work for you at lunch?"

"It seems like protein [vegetables, fruits, or a specific food] are coming back home from lunch. What new protein [vegetables or fruits] could we try instead?" or "How can we change things to make the protein [vegetable or fruit] better?"

"Tell me what you see [hear, smell, or feel] with the veggies [or other food] we've been packing for lunch. What would help it?"

On this note, invite your child to help pack their lunch, regardless of their age, because kids' consumption of food correlates with ownership in creating meals (DeJesus et al. 2019). Toddlers and preschoolers can put veggies into containers. Elementary-aged kids can use safety knives to cut fresh produce, and kids of any age can help make a sandwich or fruit-and-yogurt parfait. The key is to have your child prep or pack items *from the category of food they usually skip*. If vegetables come back home untouched, put your child in charge of packing them. For example, say, "Which new way can we make carrots?" Show them appealing pictures of that food online or in a cookbook to get ideas. Maybe it's worth ten dollars for a crinkle cutter or veggie spiralizer to up intrigue. It's not gadgets that matter, though. New table talk is what gets your child involved, lightening your load of trying to make enticing-enough meals. Tweaks made to food shouldn't be all on your shoulders, because that rarely gets kids trying new things.

New table talk supports your child experimenting with new foods. As you try new ideas, ask your child, "How's it been seeing [smelling or touching] tofu [or whatever food they tend to avoid] in your lunch? For foods that still come home untouched, use a reflective statement. Taking the same example, say, "It seems like the tofu in your lunch still needs help." Then ask an open-ended question like, "What are you noticing with tofu?" or "What would help it?" Keep this dialogue going day by day as you and your child shape things up in their lunch.

How to Respond to Complaining

Say you've been using new table talk for a while now, but the truth is your child stills whines about food. It's part of being a kid. If it seems like things are only getting worse, despite applying the Table Talk Method, it may be time to disarm the word "too" when kids complain about food or, for that matter, when they respond to your open-ended questions. As an example, picture your child painstakingly removing some ingredient they don't want from a food. Maybe they're picking out flecks of tomato barely discernable to the human eye, saying, "I don't want tomatoes! NO tomatoes!"

Imagine yourself using new table talk in this scenario. You say, "Tell me about tomatoes for you" or "What do you notice about tomatoes?" Your child's answer at this point may be that food is *too* something. For example, your child says the tomatoes are "too seedy" or "too squishy." What are you supposed to say then?

Remove Too-Statements

When your child says a food is too this or that, respond using a reflective statement, parroting back what they said but removing the word "too." So if your child says tomatoes are "too seedy," you reply, "You're noticing seedy." Literally repeat what your child said minus the modifier "too." Then ask an open-ended question like "What else?" or "What would help that?" All together it sounds like this:

Parent: How are these tomatoes for you?

Child: Too seedy.

Parent: So you're noticing seedy. What else?

Alternatively, you could respond to "Too seedy" with "So you're noticing seedy. What would help it?"

This table talk revision might seem pointless at first. How can a reflective statement (minus the word "too") and an open-ended question help a kid who doesn't want tomatoes? This tiny change works by preventing the three things that usually happen in this situation: ignoring, arguing, or acquiescing to whatever kids say is too this or that. Ignoring your child's *too-statement* means you forfeit a chance to nurture gastronomic intelligence. Arguing with their comment turns your kid off even more with that food, and validating or yielding to what they say renders that food impossible to eat.

Removing the word "too" clears the way, so the focus stays on the adjectives your child observes with this food. This allows you and your child to lean into gastronomic intelligence. "Seedy" or "squishy" describes your kid's senses coming into contact with tomatoes. That's an experience happening in their body below the eyebrow line. Well done! You're on the workable edge of this food struggle, guiding your child to use their internal compass and work with you to solve the problem. The word "too" interferes with all that. It indicates the experience is kind of intense. But discord can be downgraded when you and your child come together around "seedy" and "squishy."

Seedy and squishy foods and feelings (and *all* their counterparts) aren't something your child wants. But when they show up, opposing them only leads to more problems. Take away the word representing the overwhelm, and you gain the chance to connect with your child in the narrow margin where better outcomes are possible. Even when your child says a food is "too gross!" you can simply reply with a reflective statement stripped of the word "too." Say, "For you, this feels *gross*." (Use whatever adjective your child uses.) Your reflective statement tells your child you are listening. This helps them settle down. Now you can ask an open-ended question. Here's what to say next:

"Where's that feeling in your body?"

"How can we loosen [or change, shift, improve, fiddle] with that?"

"What's left to explore?"

"What would help it?"

The Table Talk Method for dealing with kids' fussing about food is to make a proverbial sandwich out of new table talk. Two open-ended questions are the slices of bread, and one reflective statement is the filling (hold the *too*). When your child complains or picks X out of their meal, start with an open-ended question. Say, "Tell me what you're noticing with X?" If your child says, "It's too Y," spit that back in the form of a reflective statement without the word "too." Say, "So you're noticing Y." Then ask another open-ended question like "What else?" or "Where's that feeling in your body?" or "What would help it?" You can also say,

"What can we change so X feels [or smells, looks, or sounds] better for you?"

My client Rose uses this method with her five-year-old son, Charlie, daily. "What do you notice about rice?" she asks as he pushes it around on his plate. "It's too crumbly," Charlie replies. So Rose says, "It's crumbly for you. How could you bring smooth to that?" Charlie quietly considers, then names mango as something he'd like to add on. Suddenly a small slab of fruit becomes his utensil. He presses mango into scattered grains of rice until they stick to the surface, which to his mind and palate affords a more tolerable bite. If Rose didn't have mango, she would use a different adjective or suggest another smooth food option like avocado or canned peaches. New table talk frees Rose from having to come up with all the answers. She's not fixing the rice problem alone. She's got better language that enlists her child's help, and they work through the challenge together.

Facilitating Cooperation

New table talk turns up solutions you can't imagine on your own. It facilitates true cooperation. Your words meet your child in their food discontent with new ways to sort things out instead of old ways of stuffing them down. Even when new table talk doesn't reveal a hidden fix, it speaks to and honors your child's awareness and process of eating, which is more important than keeping tabs on what they eat.

Your commitment to new table talk assures your child's gastronomic intelligence is prioritized, because that's what it takes to raise a healthy eater. Removing the word "too" is not about downplaying the significance of your child's sensory experience but about acknowledging their observations and helping them figure out how to handle it when food is displeasing for them. Big feelings come up around eating for people of all ages. And too-statements are a cue for you as a parent to guide your child gently inward—toward, not away from, their lived experience with food.

Using new table talk when kids gripe about food also lowers stress for you. To see this, ask yourself what you used to say to your child when they complained about food. My research shows parents say things they hope will make kids stop bellyaching, like "You don't need to announce what you don't like" or "You can't just say dinner is gross." There's also the cheery version: "Your taste buds are always changing. You might like tomatoes now." Is it just me, or do you feel annoyed every time you utter those phrases? They never work. And they never will. Now you can let them go in favor of new table talk. Having a plan for what to say means you won't keep getting snagged.

Drop the Four-Letter Words of Feeding

We've come to the final phase of revising your table talk. It's dropping what I call the *four-letter words of feeding*. The words "just," "need," "some," and "much" are old table talk remnants that lead to undesirable outcomes. They imply judgment, initiate bribes, and strong-arm eating situations. To hear how these words cause trouble, imagine your child declaring "I'm not hungry" or "I'm done" when they've eaten less than you'd like. How might you respond?

EXERCISE: Identify Old Table Talk

Grab a pen to complete this quick task. Read this list of old table talk responses, and circle every instance you see "just," "need," "some," and "much."

"How much of that did you eat?"

"Just try some."

"Have some more squash."

"You just need to take three more bites."

"You didn't eat much."

"What about just a little taste?"

"You don't need more bread."

"You've had too much pasta. You need to eat some veggies."

"How much pizza have you had?"

Those four-letter words of feeding show up thirteen times. Did you find them all? Before we discuss why these words are problematic, how do you feel about those responses to "I'm done?" What's your gut reaction to these examples of old table talk? Write about this in your journal if you like.

At this point in table talk training, many people say old table talk makes them cringe. If the phrases in the exercise felt unsavory to you, that's a good sign! It means your mindset is shifting as well as your words. You understand how important it is to keep kids curious and connected with their experiences of eating, and "just," "need," "some," and "much" do the opposite of that.

Why These Words Are Problematic

The four-letter words of feeding signify a lane violation in Satter's division of responsibility in feeding. Remember, your child decides whether to eat what's served and how much. When you use these words, you've probably crossed a line into territory that's not your domain, but recognizing that means you can change it. When you hear yourself say "just," "need," "some," or "much" in your table talk, pause right away. Then ask yourself, *What do I want my child to do, know, or change about their eating right now?* Take your answer to that and turn it into an open-ended question without using those four words. So instead of saying "How much of that did you eat?" ask, "Where's the full feeling in your body?"

Reread those last two questions out loud, and imagine someone saying them to you. Which phrase empowers you as an eater? Which one makes you feel judged? The old table talk ("How much of that did you eat?") is a prove-it question laden with distrust, but the new table talk ("Where's the full feeling in your body?") is born out of genuine curiosity. Can you hear and, more importantly, feel the difference? This is how new table talk improves your child's health, of body and mind, while they eat.

To cut these words out of your table talk, focus on one word at a time. Listen to what you say during meals to hear which of these words comes up. Once you identify which word is most common for you, dedicate one week to avoiding that word while you eat with your child, like a game of table talk Taboo. When you catch yourself using the word you're trying to quit, write that table talk phrase down, because getting it on paper helps you spot patterns or situations where this word consistently comes up. If your table talk is already free of "just," "need," "some," and "much," stay alert for these four words when eating with your child.

As practice, when your child says they're full, don't doubt them. Especially not out loud. And if you doubt them in your mind, don't let that seep into your table talk. This means you won't say, "You had the tiniest piece. You need to take another bite" or "Please just eat what's on your plate; it's not that much" or "Everyone who eats some, gets dessert."

As "just," "need," "some," and "much" fade from your table talk, you need other things to say instead. This next batch of new table talk trains you in something significant: how to talk to your child about their hunger and fullness.

How to Talk to Kids About Hunger and Fullness

The Table Talk Method has specific ways of talking with kids about their hunger and fullness, which might be different from what you think. For example, I don't recommend you say, "Check in with your belly" or "How full is your tummy?" Because hunger and fullness show up in the body in many places besides the stomach. I also discourage questions like "Is your belly happy?" as it's a closed-ended question that asserts emotions (like happiness) are tantamount to feeling full.

Hunger and fullness are signals observed with your eyes, nose, mouth, ears, hands, heart, mind, and more. Hunger and fullness can be felt as readily and competently in any of these places as they can in the belly, especially when you're a kid. New table talk, informed by gastronomic intelligence, broadens how and what you ask your child about hunger and fullness to include the various ways and places these cues show up.

Remember Bays's concept of the nine types of hunger? (Review chapter 5 if needed.) Now I'll show you how to apply that understanding to create new table talk about both hunger and fullness. This helps you and your child figure out which types of hunger are happening and how much hunger and fullness are present, in any given moment. You might be surprised by how much your child intuitively knows on this topic.

USE NEW TABLE TALK TO TALK ABOUT FULLNESS:

First let's talk about what to say when your kid says they're full (even if they barely ate a thing). When your child says, "I'm done" or "I'm full…" use this new table talk:

"Where's the full feeling in your body right now?"

"Locating fullness, where are you sensing it?"

"Which part's feeling full?"

"How full are your eyes for this food?" Or you can ask, "How full is your nose [or mouth, stomach, mind, or heart] for this food?"

"Feeling for fullness in your body, where is it right now?"

"What's helping you feel full?"

"How does full feel in your body?"

"What else helps you feel full?"

The table talk method for asking kids about their fullness prompts them to be aware of their five senses below their brow while they eat.

USE NEW TABLE TALK TO TALK ABOUT HUNGER

The flipside of kids claiming they're full is when they ask for food again ten minutes later. This situation is a breeding ground for old table talk, and what often gets said compromises how kids discern hunger and fullness while making everyone feel rotten. When your child pleads, "But I'm still hungry…" don't use these old table talk phrases:

"Remember how you didn't eat very much at dinner?"

"This is why I asked you to eat more earlier."

"Next time, please eat your food, so you won't be hungry later."

"I'll give you a snack tonight, but we're not going to keep this up."

Can you hear how old table talk zaps kids' chances to get familiar with hunger and fullness? When you face this predicament, talk about hunger using the same style of table talk you used to talk about fullness:

"Where do you notice the hungry feeling?" or "Where is hunger showing up in your body?"

"Where's the hungry feeling right now?"

"What part feels hungry, your eyes [or nose, mouth, stomach, heart…]? What would satisfy that? Looking [smelling, touching, hearing, imagining…]?"

"What kind of hunger is here now? What smell [flavor, texture, color, temperatures, sound, or feeling] might satisfy that?" Fill in the blank with whatever sense seems appropriate in the moment.

New table talk gets kids discerning hunger and fullness in a comprehensive way using their eyes, nose, mouth, ears, hands, heart, and mind. I know these questions might sound strange, but give them a try, even for yourself, because they're the most accurate way to sense hunger and fullness playing out. Plus this new table talk allows your child to take agency as an eater while it saves you from more squabbles.

When your child claims, "I'm full," new table talk means you don't have to cut a deal; instead of bartering with your child (*just, need, some,* and *much* lingo), you ask, "Where's the full feeling in your body?" This puts you in the role of active listener instead of micromanager of food. It's language that guides your child to sense fullness using their built-in tools (five senses, nine types of hunger, and gastronomic intelligence). These skills are useful for every meal and snack of their life! So, try these new questions and really listen to what your child says. They might be full in their eyes, nose, mouth, belly, or wherever.

When they share how or where fullness is showing up for them, reply with an ING-verb. For example, when your child says, "My eyes are full for celery," you say "Honoring that feeling in your eyes" or, shorter, "Going with that." When they say, "My mouth is all done with celery," your new table talk is "Following that feeling in your mouth" (or nose, stomach, eyes, hands, or heart, wherever they're recognizing fullness). The only thing left to say then is an ING-verb phrase inviting your child to end their meal. Say, "Clearing your plate, please."

Wait, did we just let a kid off the hook with eating because they said, "My mouth isn't hungry for this food?" That seems nuts! If you think your kid will never eat anything if you talk like this, test these questions out with your child. Ask, "Where's hunger showing up in your body?" Then listen carefully to what they say. Use their observations to formulate open-ended questions. Say, "What would help the celery for your eyes?" (Or refer to nose, ears, mouth, hands, or whatever is relevant.) Maybe they choose an add-on, or maybe their answer has nothing to do with food. Kids come up with amazing insights from the liberty of new table talk. And developing awareness of hunger and fullness can only happen with regular practice. Old table talk shuts that process down, but new table talk is a hub for its development.

TO SERVE OR NOT TO SERVE (A SNACK)

So your child said they were full, then doubles back asking for more food. You've got new table talk to respond to their request, but we've come to a fork in the road. You're either going to offer an impromptu snack or not, and you need to know what to say. If you offer the snack, new table talk consists of adjectives plus an open-ended question. If you don't serve the snack, new table talk is one factual statement and a time estimate for their next snack or meal. I've put examples of these new table talk options into a chart according to whether or not you offer the unplanned snack. Details on implementing either option follow.

Table Talk Options for Ad-Hoc Snack

If you serve the ad hoc snack:	If you don't serve the ad hoc snack:
"We have [adjectives describing foods]. What works for you?" "Your options are [adjectives describing foods]. What's calling to you?"	"The kitchen is closed right now. We'll eat again after soccer [or upcoming activity or event]. "We're done eating for now. We'll eat again at six o'clock."

If you serve unplanned snacks after meals, remember two things. You're in charge of what gets served, and leading with adjectives can help, especially if you often get stuck bargaining with your child about what they want to eat. Avoid that ordeal by making adjectives your table talk front-runner. For example, if you're offering a banana or toast say, "We have soft and sweet or crunchy and dry. Which sounds best to you right now?" This new table talk invites your child to sense into their hunger and use gastronomic intelligence to decide what will satisfy them in the moment. If the adjectives you list don't match what your child wants, you say, "Those are the options right now."

The first few times you try this approach, your child might be confused or even ticked off. They want to know what food you're offering, and you don't need to withhold that information. Just avoid leading with "You can have a banana or toast." Naming the food doesn't spark your child's GI, and it can start an argument. You know the one, "But I don't *want* a banana…" Adjective-forward table talk doesn't prevent your child from objecting. However, it gets you out ahead of that by describing food according to the characteristics they need to call upon gastronomic intelligence. This orients both of you to what matters when eating: the inward experience. It's another way new table talk teaches your child skills of healthy eating. In this case you're guiding them to choose food using mind-body awareness instead of opening the cupboard or fridge to see what's lying around.

On the other hand, if you're not serving a snack, you can say, "The kitchen is closed" or "We're done eating for now." Follow that with stating the time they'll eat next. Customize this so it makes sense to your child if they don't tell time yet. For example, "We're done eating now. Snack will be after music class." The more you practice this new table talk, the easier it gets.

Changing how you talk about hunger and fullness can be a lot to digest. For some parents it's the hardest and most awkward new table talk to pick up, because the old stuff can be really entrenched. Be patient and forgiving with yourself as you try to let go of old table talk on these themes. On the upside, you and your child get hungry and eat many times a day, and each of those moments is a fresh chance to practice using new table talk questions. Speaking of tough things to shake, it's time to discontinue the try-bite, if you're ready to say good-bye.

Getting Rid of the Try-Bite

You might have noticed how none of the new table talk you've learned makes your child taste food. That puts some parents on edge. They're not convinced their child will make progress as an eater if they don't make them try foods. One-bite rules are a polarizing topic, and I'm not here to judge. You must do what works best for your family. That said, if making kids taste food isn't going as well as you'd like—if it's adding tension to meals or setting up conditions about eating you're uncomfortable with—you can stop the try-bite. There's new table talk for that.

Dropping the try-bite involves replacing words that invoke it (old table talk) with new table talk. To put an end to try-bite rules, start with this new table talk question: "What's happening for you with X?"(X is the food your child avoids.) Ask this with genuine curiosity in a lighthearted tone (not prove-it style). You're not asking your child to answer for their disinterest but aiming to hear what's going on with their senses. This open-ended question doesn't oblige your child to *do anything* with X, which makes them more likely to explore. Their senses are at the helm. Replacing mandates with curiosity and connection is the best way to unlock new potential. Extend wonderment through new table talk; then sit back and let your child experience food.

When retiring the try-bite, ask yourself, *How much can I learn about how my child experiences X?* Go after that with open-ended questions about color, feel, smell, texture, temperature, and flavor of food. Don't say, "How does X taste?" because taste is an unwanted verb. As previously mentioned, "flavor" is a better word because it encompasses temperature, smell, texture, and taste. Focus on the other options and skip the word "taste." It's an action step your child is no longer required to take.

If you're on the fence about the merits of the try-bite, consider this: making your child try a food doesn't increase the likelihood they'll want it, like it, or eat it again later. In fact, it can do the opposite. A study of 4,845 mother-child dyads (kids age one to six) found parental pressure to eat increases children's fussy eating behavior for several years (Jansen et al. 2017). This makes new table talk even more valuable. "What's happening for you with X?" is more effective in both the short and the long run. You might be used to saying "It's okay not to like it, but please try one bite," but accumulating a series of one-off tries isn't what it takes to build healthy eaters. For more ideas of what to say when breaking up with the try-bite for good, consult the right-hand column of the "Say This Instead" chart in chapter 6.

This concludes the final piece of table talk learning! We've covered a lot of ground in this chapter, so you may want to pick one or two new phrases and use them repeatedly until they feel like your native language around food. It can also be helpful to zoom out and remember why you're doing this work in the first place.

Self-Reflection Journaling

Turn to your very first journal entry where you named things you hoped would change about eating for your child. This was part of the "Defining Healthy Eating" exercise in chapter 1. Find and read your answers to questions four and five in that exercise. Then turn to a new page in your journal, and respond to the following:

- What did you hope would improve about your child's eating?

- What new table talk do you use today if or when this situation arises?

- How does new table talk affect you and your child in terms of this challenge?

- What stressed you out with feeding your child when you started reading this book?

- How do your new table talk practices affect these feelings today?

Meeting struggles over food with greater awareness and flexibility is your way now, and hopefully you're seeing perceptible results using the Table Talk Method.

Letting go of "why," "too," "just," "need," "some," and "much" initiates new ways of cooperating with your child over food. You've accomplished that and acquired a full menu of new table talk to help your child sense hunger and fullness. This is a major component of what it takes to be happy and healthy with food! You're the best person to train your child to trust themselves as an eater, and your new words speak directly to the heart of how your child develops and practices these skills.

Next, we'll troubleshoot common bumps in the road like what to do when you "mess up" and how to deal with family and friends who use old table talk.

CHAPTER 9

Ending Meltdowns Is a Family Matter

New table talk is like a utensil, albeit an invisible one. You don't eat soup with a knife or steak with a spoon, and so it is with new table talk. You want the best tool for each situation. Figuring that out takes practice and patience, and for some people it causes a short-term problem: hyperconsciousness of how easy it is to "mess up."

In this chapter we'll cover what to do when you use table talk you wished you hadn't. I'll help you find your voice and give you pointers about when to keep quiet. We'll also discuss what to say when other people in your child's life don't know or care about new table talk. You'll meet Paul, whose partner didn't believe in new table talk, and I'll share how Paul and his partner found a unified voice. We'll end this chapter by taking stock of the numerous changes you've made.

Mistakes Are Part of the Process

Old table talk will still slip out even though you're "new table talk trained." I'm thirteen years into being a mom (the mom who developed this method), and I still say things to my kids I wish I hadn't over food. When that happens, I say, "I take that back" or "That's not what I meant to say," and then I rephrase it in a new table talk way. You can too.

Such redos are an essential part of the Table Talk Method, because table talk isn't something you can perfect. You aren't failing even if you use table talk redos every single meal. When you hear yourself say things like "What vegetables did you eat this week?" or "I think your eyes are larger than your stomach!" just pause. On the spot. Then say, "That's not what I meant." After acknowledging you want to say things differently, rephrase your comment or concern using one of the new table talk formulas from chapter 7. Say what's on your mind in the form of an open-ended question, reflective statement, ING-verb, or combination thereof.

So "What vegetables did you eat this week?" gets changed to "That's not what I meant. I'm wondering what you noticed about the veggies we had this week?" You took a prove-it question about a lack of vegetable intake and changed it to an open-ended chance for your kid to say what's working and what's not with veggies. I know this sounds oversimplified on paper, but if you don't ask this question, you're caught in the revolving door of *trying to make your kid eat vegetables.* For another decade or so.

New table talk might not excite your kid about vegetables, but it gives you a chance to say, "What would help the veggies we're having?" or "What else could we try?" or "Which green [red, orange, or purple] vegetables should we put on the menu this week?" These aren't questions you only ask once. They're your new way of communicating. When you ask your child about their observations of food, you teach them to value their experience. Not to drop out of the process because certain foods aren't compelling (yet).

New table talk shows your child that unfamiliar foods aren't things to dismiss and that pleasure is a big part of eating worth the effort of sorting out. More delight and less disgust with food don't suddenly occur when or because kids grow up. These things take proper encouragement, enough wiggle room, and lots of opportunity to practice. New table talk delivers these things. Old table talk just rams the stuck spots. It doesn't help kids learn to eat better. New table talk takes things like veggie-avoidant behavior in a different direction, so your child gets to know food and a whole bunch of new ways of relating to it. That flexibility is the output of your mindful communication.

The other example of old table talk to redo is "I think your eyes are larger than your stomach." You can change that phrase to "That's not what I meant. Choosing how much food to take takes practice. Starting small and adding more later might help. What do you think?" Alternatively, for older kids say, you could say, "I take that back. Taking an amount of food that matches your hunger takes practice. Starting small and adding more later sometimes helps. How does that sound based on your experience?" In this example, old table talk about taking more food than your child can eat gets transformed into ING-verb suggestions followed by an open-ended question.

Reread these alternatives to old table talk aloud as you imagine saying these words to your child. Can you hear how new table talk removes shame and blame while offering a clear description of something your child can do going forward to work on "the issue"? In the second example, you want your child to stop piling up more food than they can eat. Old table talk sometimes shames kids for not knowing how to decide on proper volumes of food. That really stinks, because figuring out how much food to take (or eat) is hard, even for adults! This highlights how beneficial new table talk is for guiding your child's skill development as an eater. It normalizes the guesswork and guides kids with practical tips for gauging how much food they want or need. Old table talk aimed for the same thing but struck out by making kids feel inept.

You're clued in about old table talk now in ways you weren't before, but it still takes time to leave the old stuff behind and use new language consistently. Even with a boatload of new table talk, you'll still get irritated by things your child says, does, eats, or avoids at meals. When this happens, take a deep breath. As you exhale ask yourself, *Curiosity or connection? Which can I summon right now?*

Your mindset gives rise to your table talk (old or new), which can make or break a situation. Curiosity and connection must take precedence over expecting particular outcomes, even when your child is upset about food. That means not clinging to the hope they'll eat *enough* ("Just two more bites!"), so you can back down. Instead of that old table talk, use your five senses to face the indignation. What shred of curiosity or connection can you access in your own body or mind? Put *that* into words, because it's your best shot at resonating with your child in this struggle.

Beneath all the noise of struggles over food is pure vulnerability. Picture the upset kid in front of you when they were eating in a high chair. Their basic nature as an eater is undiminished (even though this moment is infuriating). Draw upon the tenderness you used back then and speak to your child in that way. Your compassionate new table talk also recognizes this meltdown too shall pass.

When your child throws food on the floor or blows bubbles in their beverage incessantly, say six words: "What can I say about that?" This is an open-ended question for when you're totally perturbed. Its rhetorical nature gives you a minute to get it together in a new table talk way. Many parents tell me this phrase alone, when asked playfully, changes kids' behavior. But what can you say if nothing is working and the meltdown has reached a crescendo? The Table Talk Method offers a two-step plan for when things fall apart at the table.

What to Say When Things Fall Apart

Don't attempt to table-talk your way out of a full-throttle food-related tantrum. Even if you suspect your child is losing it is because they need food, STAT. If your child's on the ground kicking and screaming, they can't explore food using adjectives and their senses.

Step one when your child is totally unglued about food is to soothe them. Without using food. Comfort your child as best you can with whatever approach works for them. For some kids it's a hug. For others it's sitting on your lap or listening to music (maybe with headphones). Other kids do best escorted away from the table to ride the storm out in a quiet place. Maybe you hold their hand or send loving-kindness their way. Whatever you do, don't force them to eat. When your child's in a full-tilt meltdown, the dust needs to settle before they can eat and drink.

Step two is trying not to revert to old table talk. It's hard to choke back phrases like "Take some bites and you'll feel better" or "If you just eat [or drink] something, it will help," but those words rarely pan out. Your best option when things escalate is to say nothing at all, or to say nothing in combo with a personal meltdown mantra.

A meltdown mantra is one word you choose (in advance) to say to yourself when food freak-outs erupt. For me, it's the word "ease." I repeat this word silently in my head during intense periods of food-related distress because it helps me avoid old table talk and reminds me of my responsibility: to coach my child's inner process of eating rather than scrutinize their behavior or plate. I chose the word "ease" because it's the energy I want to bring to the hot mess I'm in. Repeating *ease* to myself calms me down and gives me enough headspace to find a shred of curiosity or connectedness. Sometimes it works. Other times it doesn't, and I fire off old table talk anyway. Then I employ the table talk redo.

When your child calms down enough to chew and swallow safely you can say, "How about something to eat or drink?" Your compassionate action and mantra of choice are two ways you can help your child through the apex of a mealtime meltdown.

Know When to Keep Quiet

Every now and then, you'll ask "What do you notice?" one too many times and end up on the receiving end of "I just DON'T LIKE IT, okay?!" When your attempts at new table talk blow back in your face, be quiet. Sometimes saying nothing is the best table talk of all.

Being silent is the hardest part of the Table Talk Method for me, but over the years I've learned how useful table talk lulls can be. When you get the urge to offer advice to your kid about how or what they're eating, try saying nothing first. Don't comment on their food or eating behavior for a solid two minutes or longer if you can. This pause gives you time to consider what to say, so it's in line with your parenting values around food. Pausing intentionally increases the odds your words will come out as new table talk.

You may even find in certain situations that a wordless message works best. Many of my clients take what they've learned about curiosity and connection in the Table Talk Method and apply it in the form of mindful action, which sometimes speaks louder than words. One of my clients has a ten-year-old who sits all folded up while he eats. His feet are flat on the chair with his knees pressed up to his chin. This posture drives his mom bonkers. She tried new table talk (ING-verbs) like

"Stretching down..." demonstrating the posture she hoped he'd mimic. Then one day during an intentional table talk pause, she kindly tapped her child's knee and discovered it was more effective and compassionate than any words she'd been saying. Her *conscious decision to say nothing* allowed a new idea to come through. There's a whole range of better options you can try now that you understand the world of table talk.

Find Your Own Voice

With new language in full swing, keep adding your own personal flare. You don't need to plan your words in advance. You can use what's right in front of you: your food, your five senses, and whatever observations your child reveals. Start with an open-ended table talk phrase like "Tell me about..." or "What do you notice?" and then let the rest roll off your tongue in a way that's true to you. For example, "What do you notice about broccoli?" might sound more authentic to you as "What's up with the broccoli for you?" This kind of personalization is something I encourage you to do.

Customizing new table talk is like making a ready-to-assemble craft project with your kid. You know those kits with precut shapes and googly eyes where everyone starts with the same materials but, when the projects come together, they all look different? That's how new table talk comes to life at family tables. The formulas give you the basic structure, but it doesn't mean everyone says the same thing.

There's more than one new table talk phrase for every eating challenge you encounter, so keep practicing new table talk when eating with your child. It's the best way to figure out what works for you and your child, so you say what you mean, and truly mean what you say, to your kid about eating. This brings up a question I hear in every workshop I teach: "What if I'm the only one in my kid's life using new table talk?"

Family Matters

Once you've transformed your table talk, how do you get others on board? Most notably, how do you deal with a partner or coparent whose table talk doesn't align with yours? When people who parent together aren't unanimously interested in learning new table talk, it can be antagonistic for the adults and confusing for the kids. The same can be said when other people who have responsibility for eating with your child, such as grandparents or childcare providers, use old table talk that contradicts your approach. Many parents ask for my help getting buy in from other adults in their child's life whose table talk they fear works against what they're trying to accomplish.

This happened with Paul, a forty-eight-year-old physician and father of two elementary school kids who wanted to learn new table talk to pass down different messages than he'd received around food and eating. Paul was teased as a kid because circa 1984 baseball pants didn't work for his body. Instead of matching his teammates, he sported sweatpants from the Husky section at Sears.

Paul doesn't remember his parents' exact table talk, apart from the old adage "There are starving kids in the world, so you need to finish your plate." He does recall, however, how he felt at his family table, feelings he describes as "contradictory and impactful." Paul says, "I was told to clean my plate but then razzed for having a hollow leg. I loved most foods, so I was easy to feed but also an easy target for criticism on topics like portions and capacity."

The work of transforming table talk has been profound for Paul and his kids, but Paul's husband, Jon, wasn't so enthusiastic at first. He worried new table talk would create a situation where they "let go of ground rules at dinner," allowing their kids to "get away with never eating healthy foods." Jon doesn't put up with kids complaining about food or asking for a separate meal. Who can blame him? But he was surprised to learn he didn't have to sacrifice his standards to use the Table Talk Method.

One evening Paul and Jon's six-year-old daughter wouldn't eat her cauliflower at dinner. That's a food she usually enjoys, so everyone was a little peeved. "Please eat some cauliflower," said Jon. And when she didn't, he asked, "Why aren't you eating your cauliflower tonight?" Their daughter, used to Paul's new table talk, replied, "Dad, you're supposed to say, 'What do you notice about your cauliflower?' not *Eat your cauliflower.*"

Jon took this potshot in stride, thanks to his stellar sense of humor, but the comment led him to explore his misgivings about old versus new table talk. Jon discovered there's a way to talk with kids that's inclusive of their eating experience but doesn't water down your authority as a parent. He learned you can say, "This is what's for dinner," while still giving your child some say-so (in the form of an add-on). Jon warmed to the idea of new table talk after witnessing two things: Paul's easier time handling food turbulence and his kids' enthusiasm for this new way of doing things.

Before this, Jon hadn't thought that what he said to his kids about their eating could bring about positive change. His initial perception of the Table Talk Method was that you just listen to your child pontificate on the color, smell, and texture of foods like cauliflower. Then he tried new table talk and found it saved him time and emotional energy. He successfully maintained order at dinner and didn't get so embroiled in food drama.

Jon has been using new table talk ever since and says, "It's not giving up or giving in. It's getting on a better track." Paul and Jon each have their own new table talk, which together sets the tone for more mindful and peaceful meals. New table talk has given them a shared sense of direction and practical words for handling things that don't go to plan. But it didn't happen overnight. It took time, conscious effort, and a willingness not to force the issue when Jon wasn't keen. No matter where you're at in terms of table talk compatibility, there are a few important things to consider if or when you're hoping to get a partner or family member on board.

How to Approach New Table Talk with Your Partner

Don't try to convince your partner by telling them how bad their current table talk is—how it's sending damaging messages. Instead, keep using new table talk yourself and let the method show its own merit. Allowing your partner to observe the benefits of new table talk for themself is more effective than telling them to change their words.

Second, don't extrapolate or project themes from your personal eating history as rationale for why your partner needs to make table talk changes, because authenticity with this approach comes from knowing it on your own. If, like Paul, you feel the effects of old table talk from your own upbringing, I strongly encourage you to find support to work through those issues. Meanwhile, modeling new table talk is the best way to inspire your partner to adopt new language.

If your partner shows interest in new table talk, here's how you can help. Use your knowledge to suggest one or two new table talk phrases that specifically address a food or eating issue your partner finds irritating. You can do this right now. Which of your child's mealtime antics get under your partner's skin? What do they say to your child when this behavior happens? Now think of one new table talk phrase—an open-ended question, reflective statement, or ING-verb—they could say instead. (You may want to refer to the "Say This Instead" chart in chapter 6 or "Quick Fixes for Transforming Old Table Talk" chart in chapter 7.) Once you come up with new table talk, share it with your partner without launching into an explanation of open- versus closed-ended questions. They might not want to hear all that. Keep using your new table talk, and let your partner try out a few lines to decide for themself if the Table Talk Method is worth their time and effort.

If your partner would never read a book like this, let alone consider changing their table talk, your best bet is still modeled behavior. Don't try handing them new lines, just keep using new table talk as you parent around food and see what transpires over time. I've heard some funny stories where a partner with zero interest wound up using new table talk by way of osmosis. An important thing to know if your partner never comes on board is that you aren't cancelling each other out when one person uses old and the other new table talk. Kids get the message to turn inward from your new language - it doesn't have to be unanimous.

How to Approach Family and Friends

It's not only partners and coparents whose table talk might clash with your own. Sometimes extended family members or close friends unintentionally work against your efforts. Josie's family is a great example. She's a spunky nine-year-old kid with the good fortune of living two blocks away from her grandmother (her Nana). Josie walks to Nana's house most days after school for a long chat and a freshly baked sweet. Josie's Dad told me when we first met, "My mother shows affection by confection."

Josie's parents don't want Nana to stop baking homemade treats, but they wish she would change what she says when offering these foods. When Josie has a rough day, Nana says, "I've got *just the thing* to make you feel better." (It's whoopie pies.) Nana also says, "Cookies will cheer you right up!" or "You deserve a big treat!" which is what Josie now expects after weekly spelling tests.

Josie's parents fear Nana's table talk puts sweets on a pedestal. To them, it designates food as both a salve and a prize, and it totally ignores a big part of the "better feeling" everyone gets from being with Nana. Sure, it's her baked goods, but it's not *only* her baked goods. Nana's loving presence and way of listening are more than mere icing on the cake. It's difficult to tease these things apart for adults, let alone kids, which is why Josie's parents asked Nana to consider new table talk.

At first Nana didn't see the problem. "What's so wrong with a little sugar?" she said. "Josie's just a kid!" But a fringe benefit of learning the Table Talk Method is that open-ended questions and reflective statements are transferable skills. Josie's parents used their new communication tools to have an on-point conversation with Nana. They said, "Your homemade goodies are a joyful part of your time with Josie. We don't want that to change. We're wondering how you feel about using new words, so the food alone doesn't get all the credit for the love, care, and connection you both feel?"

Here are some similar questions you can ask in conversations with family members:

- "We know [child's name] feels your love in many ways. We don't want to disrupt how you and [child's name] connect, but we feel like different words about food might better capture the whole picture of the comfort and delight you two share. What do you think?"

- "What aspects of how we talk about food with [child's name] feel most unfamiliar [or uncomfortable or awkward] for you?"

- "What runs through your mind when you think about how we talk with [child's name] about food and eating?"

- "What questions do you have for us about new table talk?"

Nana found new table talk a bit strange at first, but as she revised her words, she discovered what she called "an attic full of things I said about food, eating, and my own body that I never realized had such negative consequences, like referring to my 'double chin and saddle-bags.'" Nana's takeaway was that new language is one way she can be a better example for Josie.

How to Talk to Other Adults Eating with Your Child

Another category of people whose table talk might be influential in your child's life are daycare providers, babysitters, teachers, and coaches. If you have a table talk issue with someone whose job involves being in your child's life, it's important to broach the subject in a sensitive and respectful manner. Here are some things you can say:

- "We talk about food and eating with our kids in a particular way. It's different from things adults commonly say to kids about food. I'd love to share more about it with you. How does that sound to you?"

- "When we eat with [child's name], we focus on asking questions—not about how much they're eating but about what they notice with their five senses and that food. We intentionally try to avoid telling them how or what to eat, and we don't make them take a bite or taste food."

- "I'm happy to share examples of what we say to [child's name] when eating at home. I'm wondering how you feel about trying some of these phrases when you're eating with [child's name]?"

- "I appreciate you being willing to try new table talk, and I'd love to hear your observations and questions in trying this approach around eating."

I work with a family who's had incredible success with their nanny, Liz, using new table talk. She cares for the two children (ages four and eight) before and after school and regularly feeds them breakfast and snacks in addition to helping them pack their school lunches. Liz is a single mom with four kids of her own (ages ten and up) and uses new table talk at home as well as with the kids she nannies. She says new table talk has also improved how she treats herself as an eater. "I don't pigeonhole or berate myself like I used to. Changing what I say to the kids about eating has made me reevaluate how I talk to myself about food." This is a ripple effect of the Table Talk Method: you strengthen your own gastronomic intelligence!

How to Refute Old Table Talk

Most of us don't have the luxury and privilege of a Liz in our lives. And even the most phenomenal teachers and caregivers sometimes send undesirable table talk messages. This starts younger than you think, and you can use new table talk with your child to refute old table talk messages when they do come up.

As an example, my colleague texted me a photo recently asking for my help. The image was her four-year-old daughter at school pasting pictures of food cut from magazines onto a construction- paper circle. The circle was divided in half and labeled "healthy" on one side and "unhealthy" on the other. On the "unhealthy" side, her daughter had glued four pictures, cookies, a cupcake, ice cream, and Twinkies; on the "healthy" side, she'd put broccoli, strawberries, and a can of soup.

This common preschool sorting activity made my colleague cringe because it directly opposed how she talks about food with her kids. She knew one collage wouldn't undo everything they say at home, but she wanted new table talk to refute the message. She asked, "What can I say when she says tells me we can't bake cookies because they're 'not healthy'?"

Here's what I suggest when this happens to you, because there seems to be a version of this project in every grade. Ask your child, "What do you notice about cookies [or cupcakes, ice cream, and so on]?" Listen to their observations: adjectives, five-senses talk, GI musings, all of it. Then offer a reflective statement followed by an open-ended question. Say, "It seems like this project has only two options for sorting food: *healthy* and *unhealthy*. How does that fit with our family's way of being with food?"

It's tempting to offer nutrition explanations, but tread lightly if you do. And make sure any teaching you provide is equally balanced with open-ended questions. Your goal is to start a conversation with your child that you can revisit over time and to rebut tabulation and judgment as primary ways of relating to food. Below is new table talk for dismantling messages about food that don't jive with your new approach. Come back to this list as often as you can, because this topic needs regular reinforcement.

- "Labeling food good or bad isn't the best idea if you ask me. How about for you?" Listen attentively to what your child has to say.

- "Categorizing food as healthy or unhealthy is a way of thinking that misses important stuff! When you have a cookie in front of you, what matters most to you?"

- "Instead of thinking about cookies as unhealthy or healthy, you can notice their flavor, how they look, smell, feel, sound, and satisfy. What's it like eating them warm right out of the oven [or dunking them in ice cold milk]? How does that compare to calling cookies 'good' or 'bad'?"

- "I'm imagining the texture of cookies, soft and gooey [or crisp and crunchy]. How is that 'healthy' or 'unhealthy'?"

- "What's your sense of cookies in your heart, mind, hands, or ears? How about cookies' smell and feel, even after you eat them?"

With this new table talk, you can reinforce for your kid that what they can sense and observe about cookies (and all foods) is more powerful and true than labeling "good" or "bad."

Relating to food and eating with new language is a simple way to honor yourself, and it's a great way to teach your child what it really means to be a healthy eater. New table talk provides a day-in, day-out kind of care and attention that benefits your whole family, whether they take it up for themselves or not. If you want other people to care about new table talk, and maybe even adopt it too, keep modeling the behavior and words you've come to. Your approach has changed a lot!

EXERCISE: Revisit Nine Principles of the Table Talk Method

To get a fuller sense of the progress you've made, consider the nine principles of the Table Talk Method first introduced in chapter 2, restated here. How confident and assured do you feel on these topics today?

1. *How I interact with my child around food is improving.* True or false?

2. *I'm more aware of what I say to my kids while they eat.* True or false?

3. *Every parent uses table talk.* True or false?

4. *I can identify table talk phrases that might be more helpful than others.* True or false?

5. My table talk comes from a place of curiosity and connection. True or false?

6. I have ideas of what to say to my child when they're struggling with food. True or false?

7. When I use table talk I wish I hadn't, I know how to do things over. True or false?

8. No one meal, snack, sweet, or table talk phrase represents the totality of how my child eats. True or false?

9. Every moment of eating with my child is a chance to start over. True or false?

If you thought *true* in response to all these statements, great! If not, no problem. Your new table talk is collaborative and forward moving, even if it feels like a work in progress. In fact, new table talk is always evolving. You're inviting your child into their own experience of eating, moment by moment, and teaching them to practice skills of healthy eating.

No single incident of table talk (old or new) makes or breaks how kids turn out as eaters. So when you slip up, you can do things over. Any moment of every meal is your chance to start again. This also means table talk your child hears from others is something you can talk about too, and offset as needed, using new table talk. The work you're doing to recognize and create new patterns is how healthy habits form.

CHAPTER 10

How Your New Skills Endure Beyond the Table

The Table Talk Method is about staying in the moment with new table talk on the tip of your tongue, using five-senses attentiveness and mindful communication so these skills become second nature in how you relate to your child while they eat. New table talk is multipurpose. It helps you deal with food conflict today and feeds the larger, more meaningful process of how your child develops as an eater. There's no guarantee kids will eat how or what you want, but your only chance to influence their habits happens in the present moment. This *is* the snack, meal, or meltdown over food where you show your child ways of being as an eater. And a big part of that depends on what you say.

New table talk puts better words in your mouth, but that's not all it takes. Your skillful use of curiosity and connectedness (even when trouble is brewing) brings a fresh perspective to family dynamics during meals. You are not trying to make your child "less picky" or to eradicate struggles over food. You are nurturing your child's gastronomic intelligence, because that's the cradle of healthy eating behaviors.

Gastronomic intelligence is your natural state of wholeness as an eater. It's not magical thinking or make-believe. It's part of who you are, the part that knows you're worthy as an eater even if you haven't felt like that in a while. GI is like the wind. You can't see or hold it, but you can feel and observe its effects. It sweeps out old ways of doing things, which is how new table talk teaches kids to be better eaters. Your new words prioritize gastronomic intelligence—in good times and bad—so your child learns a language of pragmatic and self-affirming words around food that will serve them throughout their life.

Satisfaction, Self-Trust, and Self-Compassion

The three prongs of gastronomic intelligence are satisfaction, self-trust, and self-compassion with food. These elements are important for getting your child through mealtime meltdowns, but they also drive how kids relate to food and eating over their lifetime. In a weird and seemingly backwards way, your child losing it over food gives you more raw material to work with as you help them practice satisfaction, self-trust, and self-compassion as an eater. New table talk is what makes that happen.

Satisfaction during a mealtime struggle probably sounds like an oxymoron. But when you use new table talk like "What would help it?" things shift. Your words make space for your kid's food-related disappointment rather than fight against it. New table talk facilitates mutually acceptable outcomes like "How can we get it to good enough?" or "How can we get what you enjoy about X on Y?" These words champion okayness. They teach children how to care for themselves when food is subpar (in their view). That's crucial for ending food struggles, but it also sharpens your child's eating skills in the long term, because underwhelming food isn't only a problem in childhood. Your new table talk shapes your child's inner voice, so they grow up to ask, "How satisfying is this food for me?" or "What do I want or need as an eater that I don't have yet?" I teach people to ask themselves these questions regularly, which demonstrates how new table talk will serve your child well beyond the meltdown years.

The second element of GI is *self-trust*, which grows with new table talk when your child is upset over food (or not eating how you'd like). Old table talk undermines self-trust with phrases like "Please be a good eater. You need to eat some more," "See how much your sister is eating?" or "You're almost done! Let's have a happy plate tonight." These phrases inhibit self-trust by suggesting a child's eating is disappointing, inadequate, or bad. Self-trust is stunted when kids believe someone else must tell them how eating is going or when they've had enough.

New table talk guides your child inward to share their felt sense of the struggle. This helps kids endure tough moments with food without losing faith in themselves. Your child's self-trust blossoms when you ask

"What's helping you feel full?" instead of "Did you have enough to eat?" New table talk tells your child to believe in *their own ability* with food. That's crucial for kids because it helps them grow up not doubting themselves as eaters.

Finally, your compassion during food struggles plants seeds of *self-compassion* in your child. Your reflective statements and ING-verbs (in place of instructive and corrective table talk) generate a let's-not-be-hard-on-ourselves-or-each-other attitude about food. These new words give your child the message that they have intrinsic worth and value as an eater, even during tough times with food.

Self-compassion is a practice I learned about through the work of Kristin Neff. She is the pioneering psychologist who established this field through her research, writing, and teaching. If "self-compassion" is a new term for you, read *Self-Compassion* by Kristin Neff, PhD (2011) and *The Mindful Self-Compassion Workbook* by Neff and Christopher K. Germer (2018). My understanding of self-compassion and how I apply it to eating and gastronomic intelligence is based on Neff's definition and work.

New table talk makes your child a better eater by familiarizing them with compassionate language around food. That might seem trivial, but it means your child won't find it so foreign or difficult to say kind things to themself about food and eating in the future. Your new words today give your child a head start in recognizing they deserve self-compassion as an eater. The importance of this can't be emphasized enough!

Friendly self-talk serves eaters of all ages. Imagine your child growing up with an inner voice that says *I don't need to fix how or what I eat. I am enough, just as I am.* These statements of self-compassion with food are gastronomic intelligence in action. And there's no doubt about it: self-compassion with eating is one of the most valuable things anyone can learn to practice. You can't *make* that happen for your child, but your new table talk instills a kind of inner listening that supports self-compassion taking root.

GI Fuels Healthy Eating

Parents who seek my nutrition counseling services want to help their kids improve as eaters. They want to get kids trying new foods, eating more vegetables, and eating less processed food. They want their child to "make healthy choices," enjoy food, use manners, and not overeat. Needless to say, when I introduce the topic of gastronomic intelligence, many of them look perplexed. My client Tammy said it best: "How does the ability to satisfy yourself, trust yourself, and be kind to yourself with food help kids eat healthier stuff?" That depends on how you define healthy eating. Let's revisit that now.

In the first exercise in this book, you captured your impressions of healthy eating. How has your understanding of healthy eating evolved?

EXERCISE: Redefining Healthy Eating

At the top of a clean page in your journal, write "Healthy Eating," and then record your answers to these four questions:

- How do you define healthy eating today?

- What skills do healthy eaters possess?

- What behaviors or characteristics of healthy eating are you observing in your child?

- What does your child do or say that you consider "eating well"?

Compare what you've written here with your responses to the "Defining Healthy Eating" exercise in chapter 1. How have your ideas about healthy eating changed?

Like Tammy, you may have come to this book thinking that "healthy eating" simply means choosing certain foods over others. I meet a lot of parents who want their kid eating more vegetables and less refined sugar. When parents tell me this, I ask them to describe what skills of eating they believe make that happen.

Again, satisfaction, self-trust, and self-compassion are what kids need to make healthy choices, because learning to eat well requires feeling comfortable and confident enough to want to try new foods. If you feel like this isn't happening for your child yet, practicing new table talk during meals can help them get there. Gastronomic intelligence is the inner resource we all use to branch out and evolve as eaters. You can't buy or force it. You must strengthen it from within.

Consider this from your own perspective for a minute. What's one food you detest? Something you'd *really* struggle to eat if a plate of it showed up right now. Get a clear mental picture of this food. What is its texture? Its color? How does it smell? What adjectives describe your sensory experience of this food? Hang with that.

Now imagine I'm sitting beside you, asking you to take a bite. You're repulsed, but I'm in charge, so I say nicely, "You don't know unless you try!" How true does that feel for you?

How might things change if I invited you to say what's going on for you with this food and then listened without trying to change your mind or convince you of anything? I'm not agreeing to give you different food, but I'm also not pushing away your direct experience. My questions welcome your observations, without judgment. From there, I can encourage you to troubleshoot. I can choose words that teach you to trust yourself. I can help you scout out potential solutions, only one of which is "You don't have to eat it." Your instincts as an eater aren't shrugged off, because my new table talk tells you that you're not alone mucking through this deplorable meal.

When it comes to food, you can talk to your child from a place of superiority and skepticism or a place of curiosity and connection. And what you say to your child about their eating reinforces one thing or another. They can learn to rate food by its nutritional value and to rate their success as an eater by how they perform or measure up. That kind of trickle-down learning happens with old table talk. Someone else is in charge, and they tell you how to stay on target with eating, bite by bite as you eat or in discussions where food gets labeled "healthy" and "unhealthy."

.New table talk turns that on its head, so kids learn how to eat using their inner resources, making healthy choices by tuning into their experiences while eating. Regardless of what they're eating, kids learn how to honor their senses, trust their instincts, and seek pleasure from food with friendliness toward themselves. They learn to know which kind of food and how much satisfies them (in the moment). That's healthy in my book. And it's what happens when gastronomic intelligence is nurtured. Kids learn to eat mindfully and enjoy food as fully as they can. They branch out and try new foods based on their intrinsic interest. They recognize hunger and fullness without being told and have an easier time navigating the ups and downs of eating. They're better eaters, built from the inside out.

The perpetual failure of old table talk is that it operates with GI in your blind spot. Old table talk is at odds with what you want to teach your child about eating. It is reactionary in nature. It puts the squeeze on kids: instructing, correcting, obliging, expecting, conditioning, praising, or failing to ask in a helpful way. That holds your child back and impedes your ability to help them grow as an eater.

New table talk makes sure your language matches what you want to teach your child about eating. It is inquisitive and responsive rather than reactionary. It originates from a place of wonder, to break up frenetic energy over food and nip meltdowns in the bud. When kids sit down to food they don't want, don't like, or don't have experience with, your mindful communication and guidance enables everyone to stick with it. The same is true for times you perceive your child to be overdoing it with food. Think about eating with your child these days. During challenging moments over food, what message does your child get from you? "Try harder," "Do better," or "Let's work together"?

New table talk shows your child that pleasure is an important part of eating and that bodily cues and senses should be acknowledged and discussed. It helps kids grasp that what's served won't always be what they prefer and establishes new norms so disfavored food doesn't mean everyone crumbles. New table talk gives your child ways to be with food that feel better than freaking out, even when what comes their way is food they aren't psyched about. Your child has never been a "picky eater." Pickiness isn't a trait to ascribe to kids. It's the product of an interaction between parents and kids around food: the very dynamic you're transforming with new table talk.

The Table Talk Method is your at-home toolkit for truly raising healthy eaters. It gives you new ways to care for the inevitable challenges at your table, because mealtime distress isn't a phase of childhood you just need to push through. It's a typical part of the parent-child relationship, and you now have better skills to handle it.

New Table Talk Begets New Self-Talk

Using new table talk with kids teaches them to say kind and useful things to themselves about food as they grow up. This is important because, as mentioned before, being a friend to yourself is an essential part of being a healthy eater. It's also important because this kind of self-compassion is all too rare. We grown-ups talk about how we eat. We judge our own habits against others, the latest fads, and all kinds of pyramids, plates, and plans. This conjecturing about food happens out loud and in our own heads. The thing about our internal food scripts is they're not usually friendly words.

I have the privilege of hearing adults describe their internal messaging around food because my clients share self-talk about eating during our nutrition counseling sessions. These deeply personal stories have taught me a lot over twenty-five years, most notably how common it is for people to feel bad about themselves with food. Here's a sample of quotes from my clients, things they say to and about themselves as eaters:

"I need to do a better job eating."

"I buy healthy food, but it just sits in my fridge."

"I want to be good. I need to eat better things."

"I just wish I could eat what I want and not feel bad about it."

"I've been so bad lately. I can't get my act together with eating."

"It's terrible, but I eat late at night. I have no idea how to stop it."

"I need to rein in my eating. I just shovel it in."

"I have cravings that don't have anything to do with hunger, and then I eat anyway."

"I just need to control myself."

"I wish I could get back on track."

"I try so hard to eat healthy, but then I blow it. All the time."

"I slack. I've gotten so lax. I guess I'm just lazy when it comes to food."

"I'm so disgusted with how I'm eating."

"I need to stick to a plan."

How do these examples of self-talk compare to what you've learned about old table talk? In chapter 3, we dissected eight types of old table talk to gain an understanding of the underlying, yet unintentional messages that language conveys. To refresh your memory, I've strung together some of the hidden messages from old table talk. Here's what they say: *You have a lot to learn about eating. You're doing it all wrong. You're bad at eating. If you just eat this, then you can have something better. You don't deserve something better, because you didn't eat the thing you should've eaten. You can't be trusted to decide things about food that are in your own best interest. You try, but somehow you just keep falling short. Shame on you for not doing a better job with eating. Just follow the plan and stick with the rules. That makes you good and worthy.*

These unintended messages from old table talk may sound eerily like negative self-talk in adulthood, but I want to be clear when making this comparison. Not everything a child thinks or feels about food—or everything an adult thinks or feels about food—comes about because of their parent or caregiver's table talk. Messages around food arise in myriad ways. And this makes your new table talk even more indispensable. It is the only message you can control. Your commitment to new table talk offers much-needed fortification against the deluge of unhelpful messages about food and eating in the world today.

What you say to kids about their eating not only reduces conflict during meals but also informs how they learn to talk to themselves about food and eating. New table talk teaches your child a language of pragmatic and self-affirming words. That's critical because no one is born thinking poorly about how they eat. Old table talk messages are always learned messages, which means you can unlearn them too. Your new table talk can change the tides of this for your child over the long term.

Growing Up with New Table Talk

Growing up with new table talk is growing up as a healthy eater. You are teaching your child to ask, "What do I notice with this food?" or "How does X look [smell, feel, or sound] for me?" Your use of adjectives and five senses–based eating guides them to assess "Where's hunger showing up in my body?" and "How full are my eyes [nose, mouth, or stomach] with this food?" New table talk like "What would satisfy me in this moment of eating?" or "How could I use it later?" become near automatic in your child's process of eating.

Those new table talk phrases are just a small sampling of the new table talk collection you've amassed. Your child absorbs what you say while they eat, so keep using new table talk with intention! You'll avoid meltdowns and serve your child's highest wisdom as an eater: their gastronomic intelligence.

A client recently asked me if new table talk has a generational effect. I don't know, but I suppose it could, as most parents tell me they never thought about table talk before we met. They just said whatever came to mind, often repeating history even if they weren't proud of it. If new table talk changes how kids relate to food, it's possible someday they won't say to their own child, "Just try some anyway" or "No dessert unless you eat some spinach." Instead, maybe they'll intuitively ask, "How's this spinach look [or smell] for you?"

The benefits of new table talk are for you and your child to discover and behold. I hope these words support you and make mealtime less anxiety provoking for everyone. Parents who use the Table Talk Method consistently report fewer meltdowns, more engagement with new foods, less stress and frustration for their child and themselves, and a newfound appreciation of their child's gastronomic intelligence. Nothing renews resolve at the table more than seeing these things flourish.

Don't worry if eating at your house isn't as hunky-dory as I've described. Ending food conflict with new table talk isn't a destination. It's an ongoing practice in present-minded awareness, conscious communication, and doing the best you can. Small improvements are what you want because those are the changes that last. Think baby steps. One new table talk phrase at a time plus your mindful awareness encourages every eater at the table to feel welcome and worthy over food.

Keep these two questions in mind throughout your child's growing-up years: First, what is your biggest priority when it comes to feeding your child? And second, how does your table talk line up with what you truly want for your child as an eater? These questions help you keep going with new talk table, which matters because every child acquires messages about food and eating as they grow up. Your new words meet the daily task of feeding kids without making anyone feel small. You might be tempted to gauge progress by how many new or colorful foods your child eats, but the real determinant of success is your connection with your child around eating: how genuinely curious you and your child can be together over food. That's the best indication you're raising a healthy eater.

Here are some final questions to remind you of how to help your child enjoy food. You don't need to answer these in your journal. Let them percolate in your head.

- Are you inviting your child to share their perspectives and experiences while they eat? Are those viewpoints acknowledged and held without judgment?

- Are you guiding your child toward gastronomic intelligence, even when things get dicey at the table?

- Have you and your child found ways to be flexible and adapt around food in a moment-to-moment manner?

- What would you say empowers your child most as an eater?

The heart of healthy eating is never about feeding kids lines. New table talk is simply a language tool to help you improve interactions with your child, so their gastronomic intelligence can shine. That's what makes food fights fall away. You don't need to shape or control how your child eats, even if you secretly hoped spiffier words might finally make them eat cabbage. Your job is to help your child explore their experiences while eating, so they learn to find their own way with food.

There's no such thing as certainty when it comes to feeding kids, which makes it imperative that you speak with intention using consciously chosen words. This ensures that your efforts to instill long-term eating habits comes from a place of awareness and nonjudgment—both of food and of your kid. Raising kids who love and respect their bodies and food demands nothing less.

I don't mean to sound grandiose, but transforming table talk can change whole lives for the better, yours and your child's. New table talk reduces tension over food while teaching your child self-care and how to believe in themselves as an eater. Eating is one of the most fundamental ways to take care of yourself, and how you talk to and about yourself on that journey has a profound impact.

Your kid won't always be a kid, but they will always be an eater. They won't always eat how or what they do today, but their eating at this moment is your golden opportunity to be present with them, just as things are. Mindfully notice one small thing arising in your own senses while you eat together. Then ask your child about that, using new table talk and wide-open ears.

Acknowledgments

Writing a book is harder than I thought, and my gratitude runs deep. Thank you to Lisa Tener for coaching me through the book proposal process. To my agent, Stephany Evans, for believing in my work from the outset, and to Jess O'Brien, Jennifer Holder, Brady Kahn, and the entire New Harbinger team for proving to me there's no such thing as a stupid question, and it's never too late to ask.

My heartfelt thanks to the clients, families, and students I've worked with over the years. Your candor and authenticity are the backbone of this book. Thank you to every beloved friend and colleague who asked, "How's your book?" Your faith and enthusiasm spurred me on when I needed it most. A special thanks to Anne Muskopf, Marie Chan, Erin Wertlieb, Jessica Berwick, Caitlin H. Kirby, and Zeenat Potia for reading and sharing feedback. True friends tell you like it is, which is invaluable as a parent and an author.

To my parents, Steven and Debra, and my siblings, Allison and Joshua, for the priceless gift of family meals in my childhood years. And to my grandparents, who taught me to appreciate homegrown food and families who farm.

My deepest gratitude to my husband Michael and our daughters, Hava and Solin, who cooked and ate many meals without me while I wrote this book. Your sacrifice, support, and patience mean the world to me. You are my best teachers and my biggest joy in life.

Ellyn Satter's Division of Responsibility in Feeding

The division of responsibility for toddlers through adolescents:

- The parent is responsible for *what, when,* and *where.*

- The child is responsible for *how much* and *whether.*

Fundamental to parents' jobs is trusting children to determine *how much* and *whether* to eat from what parents provide. When parents do their jobs with *feeding,* children do their jobs with *eating.*

PARENTS' FEEDING JOBS:

*   Choose and prepare the food.

*   Provide regular meals and snacks.

*   Make eating times pleasant.

*   Step by step, show children by example how to behave at family mealtime.

*   Be considerate of children's lack of food experience without catering to likes and dislikes.

*   Not let children have food or beverages (except for water) between meal and snack times.

*   Let children grow up to get bodies that are right for them.

CHILDREN'S EATING JOBS:

*   Children will eat.

*   They will eat the amount they need.

*   They will learn to eat the food their parents eat.

*   They will grow predictably.

*   They will learn to behave well at mealtime.

References

Bays, J. C. 2017. *Mindful Eating: A Guide to Rediscovering a Healthy and Joyful Relationship with Food*. Rev. ed. Boulder, CO: Shambhala.

C. S. Mott Children's Hospital. 2017. "Healthy Eating for Children: Parents Not Following the Recipe." *Mott Poll Report* 28 (4). https://mottpoll.org/sites/default/files/documents/022017_healthyeating.pdf.

DeJesus, J., S. Gelman, I. Herold, and J. Lumeng. 2019. "Children Eat More Food When They Prepare It Themselves." *Appetite* 133: 305–12.

Feeding America. 2018. "Child Food Insecurity." https://www.feedingamerica.org/sites/default/files/research/map-the-meal-gap/2016/2016-map-the-meal-gap-child-food-insecurity.pdf.

Gerrard, D. 2001. *One Bowl: A Guide to Eating for Body and Spirit*. New York: Marlowe and Company.

Hendrickson, K., and E. Rasmussen. 2017. "Mindful Eating Reduces Impulsive Food Choice in Adolescents and Adults." *Health Psychology* 36 (3): 226–35.

Jansen, P., L. deBarse, V. Jaddoe, F. Verhulst, O. Franco, and H. Tiemeier. 2017. "Bi-Directional Associations Between Child Fussy Eating and Parents' Pressure to Eat: Who Influences Whom?" *Physiology and Behavior* 176: 101–6.

Jordan, A., D. Appugliese, A. Miller, J. Lumeng, K. Rosenblum, and M. Pesch. 2020. "Maternal Prompting Types and Child Vegetable Intake: Exploring the Moderating Role of Picky Eating." *Appetite* 146: 104518.

Neff, K. 2011. *Self-Compassion: The Proven Power of Being Kind to Yourself*. New York: William Morrow.

Neff, K., and C. Germer. 2018. *The Mindful Self-Compassion Workbook: A Proven Way to Accept Yourself, Build Inner Strength, and Thrive*. New York: Guilford Press.

Ogden, J., and C. Roy-Stanley. 2020. "How Do Children Make Food Choices? Using a Think-Aloud Method to Explore the Role of Internal and External Factors on Eating Behaviour." *Appetite* 147: 104551.

Roberts, L., N. Carbonneau, L. Goodman, and D. Musher-Eizenman. 2020. "Retrospective Reports of Childhood Feeding in Mother-Daughter Dyads." *Appetite*. 149: 104613.

Satter, E. 1986. "The Feeding Relationship." *Journal of the American Dietetic Association* 86 (3): 352–56.

———. 2000. *Child of Mine: Feeding with Love and Good Sense*. Rev. ed. Boulder, CO: Bull Publishing Company.

Sole-Smith, V. 2018. *The Eating Instinct: Food Culture, Body Image, and Guilt in America*. New York: Henry Holt and Company.

Tsabary, S. 2017. *The Awakened Family: How to Raise Empowered, Resilient, and Conscious Children*. New York: Penguin Books.

Zervos, K., M. Koletsi, M. Mantzios, N. Skopeliti, G. Tsitsas, and A. Naska. 2021. "An Eight-Week Mindful Eating Program Applied in a Mediterranean Population with Overweight or Obesity: The EATT Intervention Study." *Psychological Reports*, first published online February 14. https://journals.sagepub.com/doi/10.1177/0033294120988104.

Stephanie Meyers, MS, RDN, is a registered dietitian nutritionist and founder of Families Eating Well, a nutrition practice training parents to coach healthy eating habits in kids. She is nutrition coordinator in The Zakim Center for Integrative Therapies and Healthy Living at Dana-Farber Cancer Institute, and a former instructor in the graduate nutrition department at Boston University. She presents seminars worldwide on mindful eating, family nutrition, and cancer survivorship.

Foreword writer **Carla Naumburg, PhD,** is a clinical social worker and author of three parenting books; including *Ready, Set, Breathe* and *How to Stop Losing Your Sh*t with Your Kids*.

Real change *is* possible

For more than forty-five years, New Harbinger has published proven-effective self-help books and pioneering workbooks to help readers of all ages and backgrounds improve mental health and well-being, and achieve lasting personal growth. In addition, our spirituality books offer profound guidance for deepening awareness and cultivating healing, self-discovery, and fulfillment.

Founded by psychologist Matthew McKay and Patrick Fanning, New Harbinger is proud to be an independent, employee-owned company. Our books reflect our core values of integrity, innovation, commitment, sustainability, compassion, and trust. Written by leaders in the field and recommended by therapists worldwide, New Harbinger books are practical, accessible, and provide real tools for real change.

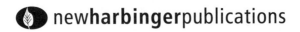 **newharbinger**publications

MORE BOOKS from
NEW HARBINGER PUBLICATIONS

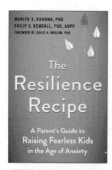

THE RESILIENCE RECIPE

A Parent's Guide to Raising Fearless Kids in the Age of Anxiety

978-1684036967 / US $18.95

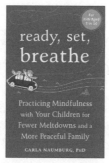

READY, SET, BREATHE

Practicing Mindfulness with Your Children for Fewer Meltdowns and a More Peaceful Family

978-1626252905 / US $17.95

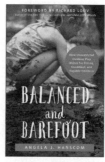

BALANCED AND BAREFOOT

How Unrestricted Outdoor Play Makes for Strong, Confident, and Capable Children

978-1626253735 / US $18.95

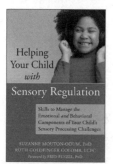

HELPING YOUR CHILD WITH SENSORY REGULATION

Skills to Manage the Emotional and Behavioral Components of Your Child's Sensory Processing Challenges

978-1684036264 / US $19.95

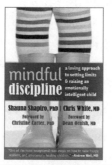

MINDFUL DISCIPLINE

A Loving Approach to Setting Limits and Raising an Emotionally Intelligent Child

978-1608828845 / US $17.95

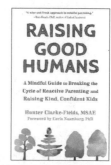

RAISING GOOD HUMANS

A Mindful Guide to Breaking the Cycle of Reactive Parenting and Raising Kind, Confident Kids

978-1684033881 / US $16.95

Did you know there are **free tools** you can download for this book?

Free tools are things like **worksheets, guided meditation exercises**, and **more** that will help you get the most out of your book.

You can download free tools for this book—whether you bought or borrowed it, in any format, from any source—from the New Harbinger website. All you need is a NewHarbinger.com account. Just use the URL provided in this book to view the free tools that are available for it. Then, click on the "download" button for the free tool you want, and follow the prompts that appear to log in to your NewHarbinger.com account and download the material.

You can also save the free tools for this book to your **Free Tools Library** so you can access them again anytime, just by logging in to your account! Just look for this button on the book's free tools page. ➜ **+ Save this to my free tools library**

If you need help accessing or downloading free tools, visit **newharbinger.com/faq** or contact us at **customerservice@newharbinger.com**.